This book is due for return on or before the last date shown below.

Sleep, Stroke, and Cardiovascular Disease

Sleep, Stroke, and Cardiovascular Disease

Edited by

Antonio Culebras

Professor of Neurology, SUNY Upstate Medical University and The Sleep Center
at Upstate University Hospital at Community General, Syracuse, NY, USA

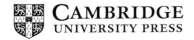

CAMBRIDGE UNIVERSITY PRESS

Cambridge, New York, Melbourne, Madrid, Cape Town,
Singapore, São Paulo, Delhi, Mexico City

Cambridge University Press
The Edinburgh Building, Cambridge CB2 8RU, UK

Published in the United States of America by Cambridge University Press, New York

www.cambridge.org
Information on this title: www.cambridge.org/9781107016415

© Cambridge University Press 2013

First published 2013

Printed and bound in the United Kingdom by the MPG Books Group

A catalogue record for this publication is available from the British Library

Library of Congress Cataloguing in Publication data
Sleep, stroke and cardiovascular disease / edited by Antonio Culebras.
   p.   ;   cm.
Includes bibliographical references and index.
ISBN 978-1-107-01641-5 (hardback)
I. Culebras, A.
[DNLM: 1. Sleep Apnea Syndromes – complications.   2. Cardiovascular
Diseases – physiopathology.   3. Stroke – etiology. WF 143]
616.2′09–dc23
2012021571

ISBN 978-1-107-01641-5 Hardback

To our patients who placed their trust in our actions
Antonio Culebras MD

Contents

Contributors

Andrei V. Alexandrov MD
Comprehensive Stroke Center, Department of Neurology, University of Alabama at Birmingham Hospital, Birmingham, AL, USA

Kristian Barlinn MD
Dresden University Stroke Center, Department of Neurology, University of Technology, Dresden, Germany

Nishidh Barot MD
Virginia Neurology and Sleep Centers, Chesapeake, VA, USA

Slava Berger MMedSc
The Lloyd Rigler Sleep Apnea Research Laboratory, Unit of Anatomy and Cell Biology, The Ruth and Bruce Rappaport Faculty of Medicine, Technion, Bat Galim, Haifa, Israel

Pietro Cortelli MD, PhD
IRCCS Institute of Neurological Sciences, University of Bologna, Bologna, Italy

Antonio Culebras MD, FAAN, FAHA, FAASM
Professor of Neurology, SUNY Upstate Medical University and The Sleep Center at Upstate University Hospital at Community General, Syracuse, NY, USA

Mark Eric Dyken MD, FAHA, FAASM
Professor of Neurology, Director, Sleep Disorders Center, University of Iowa Roy J. and Lucille A. Carver College of Medicine, Hospitals and Clinics, Iowa City, IA, USA

Alejandro M. Forteza MD
Director, Cardiovascular and Stroke Center, Jackson Memorial Hospital, Miami, FL, USA

Apoor S. Gami MD, MSc, FACC, FHRS
Cardiac Electrophysiologist, Advocate Medical Group, Elmhurst, IL, USA

Kyoung Bin Im MD
Associate in the Department of Neurology Sleep Disorders Center, University of Iowa Roy J. and Lucille A. Carver College of Medicine, Iowa City, IA, USA

Behrouz Jafari MD
Section of Pulmonary, Critical Care, and Sleep Medicine, Yale School of Medicine and John B. Pierce Laboratory, New Haven, CT, USA

Malcolm Kohler MD
Sleep Disorders Centre and Pulmonary Division, University Hospital Zurich, and Centre for Integrative Human Physiology, University of Zurich, Switzerland

Clete A. Kushida MD, PhD, RPSGT
Stanford University School of Medicine, Stanford, CA, USA

Lena Lavie PhD
The Lloyd Rigler Sleep Apnea Research Laboratory, Unit of Anatomy and Cell Biology, The Ruth and Bruce Rappaport Faculty of Medicine, Technion, Bat Galim, Haifa, Israel

Vahid Mohsenin MD, FCCP, FAASM
Section of Pulmonary, Critical Care, and
Sleep Medicine, Yale School of Medicine
and John B. Pierce Laboratory, New Haven,
CT, USA

Federica Provini MD, PhD
IRCCS Institute of Neurological Sciences,
University of Bologna, Bologna, Italy

George B. Richerson MD, PhD
Professor and Head, Neurology, Professor,
Molecular Physiology & Biophysics, The
Roy J. Carver Chair in Neuroscience,
University of Iowa Roy J. and Lucille
A. Carver College of Medicine, Iowa City,
IA, USA

**Gustavo C. Román MD, FANA, FAAN,
FACP**
Jack S. Blanton Distinguished Endowed
Chair, Director, Alzheimer & Dementia
Center, Methodist Neurological Institute,
Houston, TX, and Professor of Neurology
Weill Cornell Medical College, New York,
NY, USA

Harold R. Smith MD, FAAN, FAASM
University of California Irvine, Irvine,
CA, USA

John R. Stradling MD
Sleep Unit, Oxford Centre for
Respiratory Medicine, Churchill Hospital,
Oxford, UK

Foreword

Sleep apnea is the primordial sleep factor raising the risk of stroke to those who suffer it. That sleep apnea is a risk factor for stroke is incontrovertible and yet clinical guidelines for primary and secondary prevention of stroke remain shy if not oblivious to this fact – an incomprehensible phenomenon involving sleep disorders. Sleep apnea raises blood pressure, increases the risk of developing atrial fibrillation, alters cerebral hemodynamics, provokes brain hypoxia, increases inflammation, and does many other things to the system that eventually converge in the final common pathway of stroke. It should also be mentioned that emerging research is pointing at restless legs syndrome, periodic limb movements disorder, and even insomnia as cofactors that increase the risk of stroke.

This book aims at overcoming the clinical inertia slowing down the admission that sleep disorders in general and sleep apnea in particular are risk factors for stroke and stroke-related dementia. The book also gathers eloquent information suggesting that sleep apnea may be a factor causing deterioration of acute stroke, another phenomenon rarely considered in acute stroke units. Furthermore, sleep apnea may be delaying if not interfering with poststroke rehabilitation.

The labor of crafting a book with evidence arguing that sleep pathology and sleep apnea are risk factors for stroke would be academic were it not for the fact that sleep apnea is treatable and most of its secondary effects are modifiable by therapeutic means at our immediate disposal. Clinicians are missing the opportunity of helping their patients by ignoring that sleep apnea is a risk factor for stroke, a factor that causes acute stroke deterioration, and a factor that delays poststroke rehabilitation.

This book is intended to raise awareness of the intimate relationship between sleep and stroke. It is also a call to action for the benefit of our patients.

Antonio Culebras MD, FAAN, FAHA, FAASM
Syracuse, NY
May, 2012.

Quote

"Being sleep one of the pillars of life and one part of life marvelously full of mysteries and of symbols; being sleep the only voluptuosity that Nature offers with liberality and with same abundance to each of the human beings, the only condition being that they not be sick; the truth is that its representation in the scientific literature and in the concern of investigators is notoriously inferior to its category. Just compare what has been written about sleep and, for example, what has been written about gastric ulcers, glycosuria or asthma. This deviation is certainly strange and demonstrates that Humanity dedicates – I will not tire of saying – too much time to sleep and too little to think about its fundamental problems, among them why we sleep and for what purpose."

Gregorio Marañón y Posadillo

Speech in response to Dr. Gonzalo Rodríguez Lafora's speech of reception at the National Academy of Medicine, entitled *The Physiology and Pathology of Sleep*. Madrid, Spain; May 14, 1933.

Abbreviations

AASM	American Academy of Sleep Medicine
ACCF/AHA	American College of Cardiology Foundation and American Heart Association
ADL	activities of daily living
AF	atrial fibrillation
AHI	apnea/hypopnea index
AMI	acute myocardial infarction
Ang	angiotensin
ANS	autonomic nervous system
ARES	Apnea Risk Evaluation System
BiPAP	bi-level positive airway pressure
BMI	body mass index
BP	blood pressure
BRS	baroreflex sensitivity
BRSI	baroreflex sensitivity index
CAI	central apnea index
CNS	central nervous system
COPD	chronic obstructive pulmonary disease
CPAP	continuous positive airway pressure
CRP	C-reactive protein
CTP	computer-to-plate (imaging)
CVD	cardiovascular disease
DBP	diastolic blood pressure
DWI	diffusion-weighted imaging
ECG	electrocardiogram
EDS	excessive daytime sleepiness/somnolence
EEG	electroencephalography
eNOS	endothelial nitric oxide synthase
EPCs	endothelial progenitor cells
EPO	erythropoietin
ESS	Epworth sleepiness scale
FES	fat embolism syndrome
FMLP	formylmethionyl-leucyl-phenylalanine
HAPE	high-altitude pulmonary edema
HDL	high density lipoprotein
HF	high frequency
HIF	hypoxia-inducible factor
HOMA	homeostatic model assessment
HR	heart rate
HRR	heart rate recovery
hsCRP	high sensitivity C-reactive protein
IAD	intracranial atherosclerotic disease
ICA	internal carotid artery
ICAM	intercellular adhesion molecule

IH	intermittent hypoxia
IL-6	interleukin-6
IMA	ischemia-modified albumin
IMT	intima–media thickness
IPC	ischemic preconditioning
JNC	Joint National Committee
LDL	low density lipoprotein
LF	low frequency
LOX-1	lectin-like oxidized LDL receptor
MAP	mean arterial (blood) pressure
MCA	middle cerebral artery
MFV	mean flow velocity
MinO$_2$	arterial minimal oxygen saturation
MMSE	mini-mental state examination
MRI	magnetic resonance imaging
MSLT	multiple sleep latency test
MSNA	muscle sympathetic nervous activity
NADPH	nicotinamide adenine dinucleotide phosphate
nCPAP	nasal continuous positive airway pressure
NF	nuclear factor
NIHSS	National Institutes of Health stroke scale
NIRS	near-infrared spectroscopy
NMDA	N-methyl-D-aspartate
NOS	nitric oxide synthase
NREM	non-rapid eye movement
NTS	nucleus tractus solitarius
OA	oral appliance
OAHI	obstructive apnea/hypopnea index
ODI	oxygen desaturation index
OHS	obesity hypoventilation syndrome
OR	odds ratio
OSA	obstructive sleep apnea
OSAS	obstructive sleep apnea syndrome
oxLDL	oxidized low density lipoprotein
PAI	plasminogen activator inhibitor
PaO$_2$(CO$_2$)	arterial partial pressure of oxygen (carbon dioxide)
PD	peroxides
PFO	patent foramen ovale
PHT	pulmonary hypertension
PLMs	periodic limb movements
PLMD	periodic limb movement disorder
PLMS	periodic limb movements of sleep
PMA	phorbol myristate acetate
PMLW	periodic limb movements while awake
PMN	polymorphonuclear cells
PON	paraoxonase
PSG	polysomnography
PWI	perfusion-weighted imaging
RDI	respiratory disturbance index
REM	rapid eye movement
RES	residual excessive sleepiness

RLS	restless legs syndrome
RNS	reactive nitrogen species
ROS	reactive oxygen species
RRHS	reversed Robin Hood syndrome
SaO_2	oxyhemoglobin saturation
SA-SDQ	sleep apnea sleep disorders questionnaire
SBI	silent brain infarctions
SBP	systolic blood pressure
SDB	sleep-disordered breathing
SITT	short insulin tolerance test
SM	steal magnitude
SNA	sympathetic neural activity
SNS	sympathethic nervous system
SPARC	Stroke Prevention and Atherosclerosis Research Centre
SRBD	sleep-related breathing disorder
SRS	sympathetic skin response
SSRIs	selective serotonin reuptake inhibitors
SSRs	spontaneous sympathetic skin responses
sTNFR	soluble tumor necrosis factor receptor
TBARS	thiobarbituric acid-reactive substances
TCD	transcranial Doppler
TEE	transesophageal echo (test)
TIA	transient ischemic attack
TNF	tumor necrosis factor
t-PA	tissue-type plasminogen activators
UPPP	uvulopalatopharyngoplasty
VCAM	vascular cell adhesion molecule
VEGF	vascular endothelial growth factor

Overview of sleep and stroke

Antonio Culebras

Introduction

Even ancient physicians knew that when sleep faltered, health failed. In his famous Aphorisms, Hippocrates said "Sleep or watchfulness exceeding that which is customary, augurs unfavorably" [1]. Perhaps the statement is too general for today's usage but the concepts are immovable. Sleep is one of the pillars of health along with diet and exercise. When sleep is fragmented, not deep enough, or short in duration, a chain of events is released that leads to failing health [2]. Modern medicine has been able to disentangle some of the phenomena that disturb sleep and is beginning to foresee the consequences. Among the most notable offenders is sleep apnea, a highly prevalent disorder that incomprehensively became known just a half century ago. Sleep apnea is the term that we will use in this chapter for the generic denomination of all forms of sleep-related respiratory disturbance.

Sleep apnea alters sleep, night after night, and when so doing puts in motion a spectrum of adverse reactions that break down the physical and mental health of the individual and can lead to vascular disorders and death. The sleep apnea syndrome, that is sleep apnea with clinical consequences, occurs in 4% of adult men and 2% of adult women [3]. However, the prevalence of sleep apnea without specific complaints is as high as 24% in men and 9% in women in the general population [3]. In selected populations like the obese and the elderly, this value may be as high as 60% [4]. Furthermore, sleep apnea is not the only culprit. Recent research has unveiled some long-term vascular costs of restless legs syndrome, another prevalent condition that may disturb sleep, and is beginning to make inroads into the protracted outcomes of circadian dysrhythmias and primary insomnias.

In this book, *Sleep, Stroke and Cardiovascular Disease*, renowned authors write about the vascular consequences of altered sleep, focusing on sleep apnea, the most common and best-studied condition to date. In recent years, obstructive sleep apnea (OSA) has been identified as an independent risk factor for cardio- and cerebrovascular morbidity.

Proinflammatory risk factors

The litany of pathophysiological derangements caused by sleep apnea commences with Slava Berger and Lena Lavie's account of oxidative stress, proinflammatory vascular risk factors, and endothelial disease triggered by sleep apnea [Chapter 2]. The authors highlight the significance of oxidative stress and vascular inflammation in promoting endothelial disease and atherosclerosis in sleep apnea patients, with an emphasis on the contribution of these mechanisms to the development of cardiovascular morbidity and stroke.

Sleep, Stroke, and Cardiovascular Disease, ed. Antonio Culebras. Published by Cambridge University Press. © Cambridge University Press 2013.

Inflammation and hypoxia are intertwined at the molecular, cellular, and clinical levels [5]. Repeated hypoxia may damage the endothelium and trigger the release of proinflammatory factors like plasma cytokines, tumor necrosis factor-alpha, and interleukin-6. Chronic intermittent hypoxia causes vascular dysfunction by increasing endothelin, augmenting neurovascular oxidative stress, decreasing vascular neuromuscular reserve, reducing vascular reactivity, and increasing susceptibility to injury [6]. This state of inflammation may be related to gestational hypertension that develops in about 10% of all pregnancies [7,8] and to an increased risk for delivering preterm, small-for-gestational-age, and low birth-weight infants, along with a higher rate of preeclampsia and cesarean sections in women with sleep apnea [9].

Autonomic alterations in sleep apnea

Sleep apnea may also cause a significant increase in sympathetic activity during sleep, which in turn influences heart rate and blood pressure. Increased sympathetic activity appears to be induced through a variety of different mechanisms in sleep apnea, including chemoreflex stimulation by hypoxia and hypercapnia, baroreflexes, pulmonary afferents, the Mueller maneuver, impairment in venous return to the heart, alterations in cardiac output, and possibly the arousal response [10]. According to Cortelli and Provini (Chapter 3), sympathetic overactivity appears to be the critical link between sleep apnea and the pathogenesis of hypertension. Sleep apnea influences heart rate variability, not only during sleep but also during wakefulness. Cortelli et al. [11] showed that normotensive sleep apnea patients have a higher heart rate at rest during wakefulness and a higher blood pressure response to head-up tilt than do controls, suggesting sympathetic overactivity. When performing cardiovascular reflex tests, sleep apnea patients show significantly lower values of respiratory arrhythmia and a greater decrease in heart rate induced by cold face testing, indicating normal or increased cardiac vagal efferent activity. An increase in sympathetic activity and autonomic imbalance are possible determinants of cardiovascular comorbidity and increased mortality risk in patients with sleep apnea [11,12]. Treatment of sleep apnea with continuous positive airway pressure (CPAP) leads to a significant improvement of autonomic modulation and cardiovascular variability [13].

Blood pressure

It is known that blood pressure values normally drop by 10%–20% during sleep compared to daytime values; this phenomenon is known as dipping [14]. Nondipping, defined as less than a 10% drop in blood pressure during the night, is common in sleep apnea, and rises in prevalence as the severity of sleep apnea increases [15], as described by Barot and Kushida in Chapter 4. Nondipping has been associated with a higher prevalence of small-vessel disease and stroke [16]. In addition, blood pressure during the day tends to increase in sleep apnea patients, along with variability in blood pressure values [17]. In fact, data from various large-scale population studies clearly demonstrate a dose-dependent relationship between sleep apnea and hypertension [18,19]. Cardiologists have learned to refer patients to a sleep center for evaluation of possible sleep apnea when the blood pressure fails to respond optimally to at least three antihypertensive medications. Refractory hypertension is thus a well-known comorbidity of uncontrolled sleep apnea [20] that responds favorably to the successful application of CPAP [21]. Even children with sleep apnea may have abnormal blood pressures compared to children without sleep apnea [22] to the point that signs of cardiac remodeling, proportionate to the degree of hypertension, have been observed on echocardiography [23].

Arousal response

Dyken et al. (Chapter 5) take it one step further and report evidence suggesting that untreated obstructive sleep apnea (OSA) is a significant health risk for the development of hypertension, cardiovascular disease, and stroke. This pathophysiological pathway is mediated by hypoxemia, hypercapnia, and simultaneous elevations in sympathetic and parasympathetic activity, with significant variations in blood pressure, tachycardia/bradycardia, and asystole. The arousal response at the termination of untreated sleep apnea events conjugates many of these phenomena and emerges as a principal link in the chain of events that lead to potentiation of stroke risk factors that cause stroke.

Atrial fibrillation

Atrial fibrillation has emerged as another associated factor increasing the risk of stroke in patients with sleep apnea. The prevalence of atrial fibrillation in the United States was estimated at 3.03 million persons in 2005 [24] and has been increasing as more individuals survive into old age [25]. Compelling data have shown a strong relationship between sleep apnea and atrial fibrillation, as described in Gami's chapter (Chapter 6). Epidemiological studies suggest that sleep apnea is a risk factor for new-onset atrial fibrillation, and that sleep apnea confers a poorer prognosis after atrial fibrillation interventions. The effects of sleep apnea therapy on atrial fibrillation outcomes are largely unknown and prospective randomized controlled trials will be necessary to clarify this issue.

Patent foramen ovale

Patent foramen ovale (PFO) is very prevalent, and depending on the diagnostic method, it has been estimated to be within 10%–30% in the general population [26]. The association between PFO and sleep apnea is described by Forteza in Chapter 7. Several studies have reported the association between PFO and sleep apnea; 27% of sleep apnea patients and 15% of control subjects had PFO in one study [27]. The association of PFO and sleep apnea suggests that nocturnal apneic-related shunting from right to left through a PFO could increase the risk of paradoxical embolism and stroke. The risk increases further if pulmonary hypertension develops as a result of nocturnal hypoxemia [28]. In a study presented at the American Academy of Neurology meeting in 2011 [29], 339 consecutive stroke patients were studied. Stroke on awakening was found in 39% of patients with the association of sleep apnea and PFO, but stroke on awakening occurred in only 26% of patients if there was no association. The authors concluded that the association of sleep apnea and PFO should be considered a risk factor for stroke on awakening (OR=2.2 (CI, 1.2–3.9; P=0.01). Studies describing the association of sleep apnea and PFO are relatively few and disallow strong conclusions, at least for now. However, the evidence is suggestive and worthy of further exploration.

Stroke

Sleep apnea is also an independent risk factor for stroke. The specific risk of stroke or death in sleep apnea was investigated by Yaggi et al. [30]. In their study, the risk of stroke or death from any cause in patients with sleep apnea with a mean apnea/hypopnea index (AHI) of 35/h was expressed by a hazards ratio of 2.24 (95% CI, 1.30–3.86). The increased risk was independent of other risk factors including hypertension, while increased severity of sleep apnea was associated with an incremental risk of stroke and death.

A causal association between sleep apnea and stroke was also observed in a study in elderly individuals. Investigating 394 males aged 70–100 years, Muñoz et al. [31] found that severe obstructive sleep apnea/hypopnea (defined as an AHI of >30 events/h) increases the risk of ischemic stroke in an elderly male noninstitutionalized population, independent of known confounding factors. In another prospective analysis of 1189 subjects from the general population, Arzt et al. [32] found that sleep-disordered breathing with an AHI of 20 events/h or greater was associated with an increased risk of suffering a first-ever stroke over the next four years (unadjusted odds ratio, 4.31; 95% CI, 1.31–14.15; P=0.02). After adjustment for age, gender, and body mass index, the odds ratio was still elevated, but was no longer significant (3.08; 95% CI, 0.74–12.81; P=0.12). In a cross-sectional analysis of 1475 individuals, the same authors found that subjects with an AHI of 20 events/h or greater had increased odds for stroke (odds ratio, 4.33; 95% CI, 1.32–14.24; P=0.02) compared with those without sleep apnea (AHI<5 events/h) after adjustment for known confounding factors. The authors concluded that there is a strong association between moderate to severe sleep-disordered breathing and stroke, independent of confounding factors. In the Sleep Heart Health Study [33], men in the highest AHI quartile (>19 events/hr) had an adjusted hazard ratio of stroke of 2.86 (95% CI, 1.1–7.4). In the mild to moderate range (AHI, 5–25 events/hr), each one-unit increase in AHI in men was estimated to increase stroke risk by 6% (95% CI, 2%–10%). In women, stroke risk increased when there was an AHI of >25 events/h.

Small-vessel disease and cognitive dysfunction

Sleep apnea may also lead to cognitive dysfunction from the effects of chronic hypoxia and sympathetic stress associated with small-vessel disease in the brain, white matter ischemia, and lacunar strokes. In Chapter 8, Román reports the observation of deleterious effects of OSA on cognitive functions demonstrated in patients referred to the Alzheimer and Dementia Clinic of the Methodist Neurological Institute in Houston, Texas (Román, unpublished data). Magnetic resonance imaging (MRI) of the brain showed that OSA was accompanied by varying intensities of cerebral small-vessel disease, appearing as periventricular hyperintensities of the white matter and lacunar strokes, which would correlate with the clinical picture of subcortical prefrontal dysfunction, sometimes mixed with features of Alzheimer's disease.

In a recent publication, Yaffe et al. [34] reported that elderly women affected by OSA develop cognitive deficits when compared to age-matched controls with normal sleep. The authors concluded that cognitive decline correlated with hypoxemia rather than with fragmentation of sleep architecture caused by apneas and hypopneas. Román, along with other authors, is hopeful that early recognition and treatment with CPAP may result in improvement of cognitive function [35] and prevention of dementia in patients with sleep apnea.

Cerebral hemodynamic changes

When the cerebral circulation is compromised, hemodynamic alterations may act as triggers of irreversible ischemic changes in regions with poor hemodynamic reserve, particularly borderzone areas and terminal artery territories. Preliminary studies of auditory event-related potentials in patients with treated sleep apnea [36] found no improvement in abnormal P3 wave latencies, suggesting permanent structural changes in the white matter of the hemispheres likely as a result of ischemia. On the other hand, healthy children with mild sleep-disordered breathing [37] have cerebral hemodynamic and neurobehavioral changes that are potentially reversible following adenotonsillectomy, suggesting normalization of middle cerebral artery blood flow as measured with transcranial Doppler techniques [38].

Cerebral blood flow studies have shown that during the apnea event there is significant reduction in middle cerebral artery blood flow velocity [39,40]. The drop correlates with the duration of the apnea event rather than with the depth of oxyhemoglobin desaturation. The phenomenon suggests that hemodynamic disturbances caused by profound intrathoracic negative pressures during obstructive apneas determine a reduction of cerebral blood flow. Intracranial hemodynamic changes occurring repeatedly night after night in patients with marginal circulatory reserve may contribute to raising the risk of stroke, in particular in patients with significant sleep apnea disorder [41]. Using near-infrared spectroscopy (NIRS), Pizza et al. [42] observed that cerebral hemodynamic autoregulatory mechanisms fail with brain hypoxia in the presence of frequent apneas (AHI>30 events/h).

Acute stroke

Extending the concept of cerebral hemodynamic alterations in patients with sleep apnea, Barlinn and Alexandrov (Chapter 9) review the notions of altered vasomotor reactivity in patients with acute stroke. They report the occurrence of intracranial blood flow steal in response to changing vasodilatory stimuli like carbon dioxide elevations in patients with sleep apnea and stroke and propose that this phenomenon, termed reversed Robin Hood syndrome [43], might play a pivotal role in clinical deterioration after an acute stroke. These observations have led to the notion that noninvasive ventilatory correction in select acute stroke patients might have a beneficial effect on sleep apnea and brain perfusion and constitute a missing link in the pathogenesis of early neurological deterioration and stroke recurrence.

Continuous positive airway pressure treatment

The gold standard treatment of clinically significant sleep apnea is achieved with nightly applications of CPAP. Kohler and Stradling (Chapter 10) review the effects of CPAP treatment on stroke risk factor control and on stroke outcomes. The effect of CPAP on systemic blood pressure in patients with sleep apnea appears to depend on the severity of sleep-disordered breathing, daytime sleepiness, the extent of obesity, and the hours of nightly CPAP use. Continuous positive airway pressure treatment has been shown to decrease nocturnal arousal frequency and suppress acute blood pressure fluctuations. Randomized controlled trials have established that CPAP treatment of symptomatic patients with moderate to severe sleep apnea lowers blood pressure levels. The precise mechanism of this favorable effect remains to be identified, although there is suggestive evidence that CPAP reduces blood pressure primarily by stabilizing the sympathetic–vagal balance. Patients with drug resistant hypertension, requiring three antihypertensive drugs or more for control of blood pressure, should be screened for sleep apnea, because succesful CPAP therapy leads to significant blood pressure reductions that are greater than what can be achieved with drugs alone [44].

Continuous positive airway pressure therapy may have a favorable effect on atrial fibrillation recurrence. Preliminary observational studies have shown reduction in recurrence of atrial fibrillation following therapeutic procedures in patients treated with CPAP [45,46]. However, additional research is required to confirm this therapeutic action of CPAP.

The effect of CPAP on stroke recurrence remains to be established. It can be surmised that if CPAP exerts a favorable effect on controlling stroke risk factors, the occurrence or recurrence of stroke might be reduced. Preliminary evidence from several studies suggests that this is the case [47,48]; however, large randomized, controlled, and prospective studies need to be conducted to establish the favorable effect of CPAP on stroke occurrence.

Poststroke sleep apnea and rehabilitation

Several studies have shown that sleep apnea is common in patients after stroke [49–52]. This important observation and its implications for rehabilitation of patients following stroke is reviewed by Jafari and Mohsenin in Chapter 11. The prevalence of sleep apnea poststroke has a range of 50%–75%, depending on the study. Whether sleep apnea precedes the occurrence of stroke or appears poststroke remains a matter of debate. It may well be that both etiopathological mechanisms play a role. Sleep apnea may contribute to neurological deterioration during the acute stages of stroke and may worsen the rehabilitation outcome weeks and months after stroke occurrence. Some studies have shown that central sleep apneas predominate initially, giving way to obstructive apneas in the chronic stages following acute stroke [53].

The relationship of sleep apnea to poor functional outcome, delirium, depressed mood, cognitive functioning, ability to perform activities of daily living (ADL), as well as psychiatric and behavior symptoms has been studied in patients undergoing rehabilitation for stroke by several authors [54]. Some studies have shown that sleep apnea is significantly and independently related to functional impairment and length of hospitalization following stroke [55,56].

The feasibility and effectiveness of CPAP therapy, particularly auto-CPAP, in patients with sleep apnea and stroke have been investigated both in the acute and chronic phases [48,57,58]. Preliminary results show a beneficial effect of auto-CPAP during the acute phases of stroke [59] as well as on neurological and cognitive functions during the stable phase of stroke in a rehabilitation setting. However, compliance with treatment is a challenging proposition that needs to be resolved before this treatment becomes generalized.

Restless legs syndrome, periodic limb movements of sleep, and risk of stroke

Alterations of sleep other than those caused by sleep apnea may increase the risk of stroke. Emerging evidence suggests that restless legs syndrome (RLS) and its associated condition, periodic limb movements of sleep (PLMS), represent risk factors for cardio- and cerebrovascular disease, even leading to stroke [60–62]. This topic is reviewed in Chapter 12 by Federica Provini. Although the reasons for this association remain unclear, emerging evidence suggests that common factors prevalent in both conditions, like smoking, the metabolic syndrome, and diabetes, may predispose individuals to heart disease and stroke. However, sympathetic activation and metabolic dysregulation may constitute the common pathogenetic pathway. Repeated nocturnal heart rate and blood pressure rises accompanying PLMS, especially those occurring with microarousals [63], may facilitate development of daytime hypertension paving the way to heart disease and stroke [64]. More research is needed to evaluate the role of RLS and PLMS in increasing cardiovascular risk.

Physician as patient: a personal story of stroke

The final chapter is the personal account of a stroke narrated by Harold Smith, a renowned sleep specialist (Chapter 13). Dr. Smith suffered a disabling stroke at the height of his career as neurologist and sleep specialist. His account is most edifying and provides insights rarely retrieved from patients who suffer a stroke.

Concluding remarks

Scientific evidence linking sleep alterations, in particular sleep apnea, with stroke risk factors, cardiovascular disease, and stroke has been uncovered sufficiently well to consider sleep apnea as a strong risk factor for stroke and cardiovascular disease. Sleep apnea is a modifiable risk factor and therefore efforts to control this condition in patients at risk of vascular disease is a clinical endeavor that should be pursued vigorously, even though clinical research needs to persist in its quest to answer pressing pathophysiological questions.

References

1. *The Aphorisms of Hippocrates*. The Classics of Medicine Library. Birmingham, AL: Leslie B Adams Jr, Gryphons Editions Ltd, 1982.

2. Culebras A. Sleep and stroke. *Neurology* 2009; **29**: 438–45.

3. Young T, Palta M, Dempsey J, et al. The occurrence of sleep-disordered breathing among middle-aged adults. *N Engl J Med* 1993; **328**: 1230–5.

4. Punjabi NM. The epidemiology of adult obstructive sleep apnea. *Proc Am Thorac Soc* 2008; **5**: 136–43.

5. Eltzschig HK, Carmeliet P. Hypoxia and inflammation. *N Engl J Med* 2011; **364**: 656–65.

6. Iadecola C. *Cerebrovascular Dysfunction in Chronic Intermittent Hypoxia*. Los Angeles, CA: International Stroke Conference, 2011.

7. Champagne K, Schwartzman K, Opatrny L, et al. Obstructive sleep apnoea and its association with gestational hypertension. *Eur Respir J* 2009; **33**: 559–65.

8. Poyares D, Guilleminault C, Hachul H, et al. Pre-eclampsia and nasal CPAP: part 2. Hypertension during pregnancy, chronic snoring, and early nasal CPAP intervention. *Sleep Med* 2007; **9**: 15–21.

9. Bourjeily G, Ankner G, Mohsenin V. Sleep-disordered breathing in pregnancy. *Clin Chest Med* 2011; **32**: 175–89.

10. Somers VK, Dyken ME, Clary MP, et al. Sympathetic neural mechanisms in obstructive sleep apnea. *J Clin Invest* 1995; **96**: 1897–904.

11. Cortelli P, Parchi P, Sforza E, et al. Cardiovascular autonomic dysfunction in normotensive awake subjects with obstructive sleep apnoea syndrome. *Clin Auton Res* 1994; **4**: 57–62.

12. Friedman O, Logan AG. The price of obstructive sleep apnea-hypopnea: hypertension and other ill effects. *Am J Hypertens* 2009; **22**: 474–83.

13. Noda A, Nakata S, Koike Y, et al. Continuous positive airway pressure improves daytime baroreflex sensitivity and nitric oxide production in patients with moderate to severe obstructive sleep apnea syndrome. *Hypertens Res* 2007; **30**: 669–76.

14. Coccagna G, Mantovani M, Brignani F, et al. Laboratory note. Arterial pressure changes during spontaneous sleep in man. *Electroencephalogr Clin Neurophysiol* 1971; **31**: 277–81.

15. Hla KM, Young T, Finn L, et al. Longitudinal association of sleep-disordered breathing and nondipping of nocturnal blood pressure in the Wisconsin Sleep Cohort Study. *Sleep* 2008; **31**: 795–800.

16. Kario K, Pickering TG, Matsuo T, et al. Stroke prognosis and abnormal nocturnal blood pressure falls in older hypertensives. *Hypertension* 2001; **38**: 852–7.

17. Narkiewicz K, Montano N, Cogliati C, et al. Altered cardiovascular variability in obstructive sleep apnea. *Circulation* 1998; **98**: 1071–7.

18. Nieto FJ, Young TB, Lind BK, et al. Association of sleep-disordered breathing, sleep apnea, and hypertension in a large community-based study. Sleep Heart Health Study. *JAMA* 2000; **283**: 1829–36.
19. Peppard PE, Young T, Palta M, et al. Prospective study of the association between sleep-disordered breathing and hypertension. *N Engl J Med* 2000; **342**: 1378–84.
20. Logan AG, Perlikowski SM, Mente A, et al. High prevalence of unrecognized sleep apnoea in drug-resistant hypertension. *J Hypertens* 2001; **19**: 2271–7.
21. Dernaika TA, Kinasewitz GT, Tawk MM. Effects of nocturnal continuous positive airway pressure therapy in patients with resistant hypertension and obstructive sleep apnea. *J Clin Sleep Med* 2009; **5**: 103–7.
22. Horne RS, Yang JS, Walter LM, et al. Elevated blood pressure during sleep and wake in children with sleep-disordered breathing. *Pediatrics* 2011; **128**: e85–92.
23. Amin R, Somers VK, McConnell K, et al. Activity-adjusted 24-hour ambulatory blood pressure and cardiac remodeling in children with sleep disordered breathing. *Hypertension* 2008; **51**: 84–91.
24. Naccarelli GV, Varker H, Lin J, et al. Increasing prevalence of atrial fibrillation and flutter in the United States. *Am J Cardiol* 2009; **104**: 1534–9.
25. Miyasaka Y, Barnes ME, Gersh BJ, et al. Secular trends in incidence of atrial fibrillation in Olmsted County, Minnesota, 1980 to 2000, and implications on the projections for future prevalence. *Circulation* 2006; **114**: 119–25.
26. Lynch JJ, Schuchard GH, Gross CM, et al. Prevalence of right-to-left atrial shunting in a healthy population: detection by Valsalva maneuver contrast echocardiography. *Am J Cardiol* 1984; **53**: 1478–80.
27. Beelke M, Angeli S, Del Sette M, et al. Prevalence of patent foramen ovale in subjects with obstructive sleep apnea: a transcranial Doppler ultrasound study. *Sleep Med* 2003; **4**: 219–23.
28. Sanner BM, Doberauer C, Konermann M, et al. Pulmonary hypertension in patients with obstructive sleep apnea syndrome. *Arch Intern Med* 1997; **157**: 2483–7.
29. Ciccone A, Nobili L, Roccatagliata DV, et al. Causal role of sleep apneas and patent foramen ovale in wake-up stroke. *Neurology* 2011; **76**: A170.
30. Yaggi HK, Concato J, Kernan WN, et al. Obstructive sleep apnea as a risk factor for stroke and death. *N Engl J Med* 2005; **353**: 2034–41.
31. Muñoz R, Durán-Cantolla J, Martínez-Vila E, et al. Severe sleep apnea and risk of ischemic stroke in the elderly. *Stroke* 2006; **37**: 2317–21.
32. Arzt M, Young T, Finn L, et al. Association of sleep-disordered breathing and the occurrence of stroke. *Am J Respir Crit Care Med* 2005; **172**: 1447–51.
33. Redline S, Yenokyan G, Gottlieb DJ, et al. Obstructive sleep apnea-hypopnea and incident stroke: the Sleep Heart Health Study. *Am J Respir Crit Care Med* 2010; **182**: 269–77.
34. Yaffe K, Laffan AM, Harrison SL, et al. Sleep-disordered breathing, hypoxia, and risk of mild cognitive impairment and dementia in older women. *JAMA* 2011; **306**: 613–19.
35. Matthews EE, Aloia MS. Cognitive recovery following positive airway pressure (PAP) in sleep apnea. *Prog Brain Res* 2011; **190**: 71–88.
36. Neau JP, Paquereau J, Meurice JC, et al. Auditory event-related potentials before and after treatment with nasal continuous positive airway pressure in sleep apnea syndrome. *Eur J Neurol* 1996; **3**: 29–35.
37. Hill CM, Hogan AM, Onugha N, et al. Increased cerebral blood flow velocity in children with mild sleep-disordered breathing: a possible association with abnormal neuropsychological function. *Pediatrics* 2006; **118**: e1100–8.
38. Hogan AM, Hill CM, Harrison D, et al. Cerebral blood flow velocity and cognition in children before and after adenotonsillectomy. *Pediatrics* 2008; **122**: 75–82.
39. Netzer N, Werner P, Jochums I, et al. Blood flow of the middle cerebral artery with sleep-disordered breathing. Correlation with obstructive hypopneas. *Stroke* 1998; **29**: 87–93.

40. Netzer NC. Impaired nocturnal cerebral hemodynamics during long obstructive apneas: the key to understanding stroke in OSAS patients? *Sleep* 2010; **33**: 146–7.

41. Jiménez PE, Coloma R, Segura T. Brain haemodynamics in obstructive sleep apnea syndrome. *Rev Neurol* 2005; **41**: S21–4.

42. Pizza F, Biallas M, Wolf M, et al. Nocturnal cerebral hemodynamics in snorers and in patients with obstructive sleep apnea: a near-infrared spectroscopy study. *Sleep* 2010; **33**: 205–10.

43. Alexandrov AV, Nguyen HT, Rubiera M, et al. Prevalence and risk factors associated with reversed Robin Hood syndrome in acute ischemic stroke. *Stroke* 2009; **40**: 2738–42.

44. Lozano L, Tovar JL, Sampol G, et al. Continuous positive airway pressure treatment in sleep apnea patients with resistant hypertension: a randomized, controlled trial. *J Hypertens* 2010; **28**: 2161–8.

45. Patel D, Mohanty P, Di Biase L, et al. Safety and efficacy of pulmonary vein antral isolation in patients with obstructive sleep apnea: the impact of continuous positive airway pressure. *Circ Arrhythm Electrophysiol* 2010; **3**: 445–51.

46. Kanagala R, Murali NS, Friedman PA, et al. Obstructive sleep apnea and the recurrence of atrial fibrillation. *Circulation* 2003; **107**: 2589–94.

47. Parra O, Sánchez-Armengol A, Bonnin M, et al. Early treatment of obstructive apnoea and stroke outcome: a randomised controlled trial. *Eur Respir J* 2011; **37**: 1128–36.

48. Bravata DM, Concato J, Fried T, et al. Continuous positive airway pressure: evaluation of a novel therapy for patients with acute ischemic stroke. *Sleep* 2011; **34**: 1271–7.

49. Dyken ME, Im KB. Obstructive sleep apnea and stroke. *Chest* 2009; **136**: 1668–77.

50. Yaggi H, Mohsenin V. Obstructive sleep apnoea and stroke. *Lancet Neurol* 2004 ; **3**: 333–42.

51. Hudgel DW, Devadatta P, Quadri M, et al. Mechanism of sleep-induced periodic breathing in convalescing stroke patients and healthy elderly subjects. *Chest* 1993; **104**: 1503–10.

52. Mohsenin V, Valor R. Sleep apnea in patients with hemispheric stroke. *Arch Phys Med Rehabil* 1995; **76**: 71–6.

53. Parra O, Arboix A, Bechich S, et al. Time course of sleep-related breathing disorders in first-ever stroke or transient ischemic attack. *Am J Respir Crit Care Med* 2000; **161**: 375–80.

54. Good DC, Henkle JQ, Gelber D, et al. Sleep-disordered breathing and poor functional outcome after stroke. *Stroke* 1996; **27**: 252–9.

55. Sandberg O, Franklin KA, Bucht G, et al. Sleep apnea, delirium, depressed mood, cognition, and ADL ability after stroke. *J Am Geriatr Soc* 2001; **49**: 391–7.

56. Kaneko Y, Hajek VE, Zivanovic V, et al. Relationship of sleep apnea to functional capacity and length of hospitalization following stroke. *Sleep* 2003; **26**: 293–7.

57. Cherkassky T, Oksenberg A, Froom P, et al. Sleep-related breathing disorders and rehabilitation outcome of stroke patients: a prospective study. *Am J Phys Med Rehabil* 2003; **82**: 452–5.

58. Ryan CM, Bayley M, Green R, et al. Influence of continuous positive airway pressure on outcomes of rehabilitation in stroke patients with obstructive sleep apnea. *Stroke* 2011; **42**: 1062–7.

59. Bravata DM, Concato J, Fried T, et al. Auto-titrating continuous positive airway pressure for patients with acute transient ischemic attack: a randomized feasibility trial. *Stroke* 2010; **41**: 1464–70.

60. Portaluppi F, Cortelli P, Buonaura GC, et al. Do restless legs syndrome (RLS) and periodic limb movements of sleep (PLMS) play a role in nocturnal hypertension and increased cardiovascular risk of renally impaired patients? *Chronobiol Int* 2009; **26**: 1206–21.

61. Lindner A, Fornadi K, Lazar AS, et al. Periodic limb movements in sleep are associated with stroke and cardiovascular risk factors in patients with renal failure. *J Sleep Res* 2012; **21**: 297–307.

62. La Manna G, Pizza F, Persici E, et al. Restless legs syndrome enhances cardiovascular risk and mortality in patients with end-stage kidney disease undergoing long-term haemodialysis

treatment. *Nephrol Dial Transplant* 2011; **26**: 1976–83.

63. Pennestri MH, Montplaisir J, Colombo R, et al. Nocturnal blood pressure changes in patients with restless legs syndrome. *Neurology* 2007; **68**: 1213–18.

64. Walters AS, Rye DB. Review of the relationship of restless legs syndrome and periodic limb movements in sleep to hypertension, heart disease, and stroke. *Sleep* 2009; **32**: 589–97.

Sleep apnea, oxidative stress, proinflammatory vascular risk factors, and endothelial disease

Slava Berger and Lena Lavie

Introduction

In recent years, obstructive sleep apnea (OSA) was identified as an independent risk factor for cardio- and cerebrovascular morbidity as well as a major public health problem. Obstructive sleep apnea is characterized by intermittent and recurrent respiratory cessations termed apneas or hypopneas, which lead to blood hypoxemia, hypercapnia, and sleep fragmentation [1]. Obstructive sleep apnea is prevalent in at least 4% of adult men and 2% of adult women. However, the prevalence of sleep-disordered breathing (SDB) (without characteristic complaints) is estimated to be as high as 24% in men and 9% in women in the general population. In selected populations like the obese and the elderly, this value may rise up to 60% [2]. Moreover, SDB is prevalent in more than 60% of patients with acute myocardial infarction and in more than 50% (44%–93%) of patients with stroke [3].

A great number of clinical prospective and epidemiological studies demonstrated that the prevalence of cardiovascular associated risk factors such as hypertension, hyperlipidemia, hyperglycemia, and sympathetic activation is increased in OSA [1]. Thus, the impact of OSA on the cardio- and cerebrovascular system has been well established over the last decade and has become a recognized cardiovascular and cerebrovascular risk factor [4]. Obstructive sleep apnea is now implicated in the etiopathogenesis of stroke, coronary artery disease, and congestive heart failure. The putative mechanisms involved in the pathogenesis of cardiovascular disease in OSA include fibrinolytic imbalance, oxidative stress, inflammation, endothelial dysfunction, and atherosclerosis [4]. Moreover, evidence from the past few years suggests that the impaired endothelial function associated with OSA is largely attributed to increased production of reactive oxygen species (ROS), which promote oxidative stress and vascular inflammation. These two fundamental mechanisms participate largely in the development of endothelial dysfunction and subsequent atherosclerosis.

The present chapter will highlight the significance of oxidative stress and vascular inflammation in promoting endothelial disease and atherosclerosis in sleep apnea patients, with an emphasis on the contribution of these mechanisms to the development of cardiovascular morbidity and stroke in these patients.

Sleep, Stroke, and Cardiovascular Disease, ed. Antonio Culebras. Published by Cambridge University Press. © Cambridge University Press 2013.

Obstructive sleep apnea

Characteristics and treatment

Obstructive sleep apnea, the most common type of SDB, is characterized by repetitive oropharyngeal collapse of the upper airway during sleep, leading to pauses in respiration and subsequent arousals. Apnea is a complete cessation in airflow that lasts at least 10 seconds, and hypopnea is a partial decrease in airflow lasting at least 10 seconds. The total number of apneas and hypopneas divided by the hours of sleep is termed the apnea/hypopnea index (AHI) and is indicative of the severity of the syndrome. An AHI of >5 events/h is a widely used cutoff point between healthy subjects and patients. Apnea/hypopnea index values of 5–15, 15–30, and >30 events/h are considered mild, moderate, and severe, respectively. Although 5 events/h is the classical definition for the cutoff point [5], in more recent studies a cutoff of >10 events/h is often used to distinguish between patients with and without OSA. Complaints such as excessive daytime sleepiness, loud snoring, nonrefreshing sleep, and chronic fatigue accompanied by an AHI define the OSA syndrome. In addition, OSA can be diagnosed by the number of blood oxygen desaturations of at least 3% normalized by the hours of sleep (oxygen desaturation index, ODI) using a cutoff point of an ODI of >5. An additional parameter employed for the diagnosis of OSA and its severity is arterial minimal oxygen saturation (MinO$_2$) during the sleeping period. Oxygen saturation values below 90% are considered pathological.

Treatment of OSA with nasal continuous positive airway pressure (nCPAP) is the most effective and safe form of treatment. It helps to maintain the airway open and thus alleviates the repeated obstructions. It was stated that OSA patients with an AHI higher than 30 events/h should be treated with nCPAP. However, patients with milder OSA (AHI <30 events/h) and symptoms, such as excessive daytime sleepiness, impaired cognition, and chronic fatigue, or documented cardiovascular disease are also advised to have nCPAP therapy [4]. Significantly lower risk for cardiovascular morbidity and mortality was shown in patients subjected to successful nCPAP therapy [6].

Obstructive sleep apnea and stroke

Stroke is the most common form of cerebrovascular disease. The onset of stroke is associated with major neurological deficits, followed by acute loss of neural function due to insufficient blood supply to the brain. More than 80% of strokes are ischemic in nature, in which impaired cerebral perfusion can lead to dysfunction of brain tissue in the affected area. Narrowing of the arteries in the head or neck is the most common cause for ischemic stroke. Such obstruction of the blood vessels can be initiated by atherogenic plaque formation or cholesterol deposition in the arterial wall, leading to blood clot formation and artery blockage in the brain area [7].

As mentioned earlier, OSA was identified as an independent risk factor for cerebrovascular diseases [4,8]. A direct association between sleep apnea and stroke was confirmed by a strong adjusted correlation of the AHI with ischemic stroke risk factors and the incidence of stroke. Medeiros et al. [9] reported that OSA is extremely highly prevalent in patients with stroke. Among 50 men studied during the first week after the stroke, all had an AHI higher than 5 events/h, while 70% were diagnosed with severe OSA (AHI ≥30 events/h). In a study by Yaggi et al. [10], it was estimated that in patients with OSA, after adjusting for cardiovascular risk factors, the risk of stroke hazard ratio was 2 (1.12–3.48), and with an AHI of >36 events/h the risk was higher (hazard ratio 3.3; 95% CI 1.74–6.26). Data from a longitudinal cohort study by Redline et al. provided convincing evidence that the severity of OSA increases the risk for ischemic stroke in the male population [11]. Importantly, nCPAP treatment reduced excessive risk for mortality and for developing nonfatal cardiovascular events in patients with OSA after ischemic stroke [12,13]. It was suggested that elevated generation of ROS, release of proinflammatory cytokines, activation of the sympathetic nervous system, endothelial dysfunction, and blood pressure may contribute directly to the development of stroke in patients with OSA [3].

Oxidative stress in obstructive sleep apnea, cardiovascular morbidity, and stroke

Oxidative and nitrosative stress

Oxidative stress represents an imbalance in the cellular redox system. It has long been recognized as a fundamental mechanism underlying many seemingly unrelated pathologies by initiating atherogenic sequelae [8,14]. Oxidative stress can arise from increased production of ROS, from decreased antioxidant activity, or from both. Reactive oxygen species is a collective term used for various oxygen-free radicals such as superoxide anion ($O_2\bullet^-$), hydroxyl radical ($\bullet OH$), peroxyl (RsO2), hydrogen peroxide (H_2O_2), hypochlorous acid (HClO), and lipid peroxides. These radicals are formed as by-products of normal oxygen metabolism through mitochondrial respiration but could be generated spontaneously, or by several enzymatic reactions through NADPH oxidase, xanthine oxidase, or "uncoupled" nitric oxide synthase. The mitochondria are the leading source for cellular ROS production in most cell types and tissues.

In physiogical conditions, ROS participate as second messengers in a plethora of signaling pathways, but once the tightly regulated balance is disrupted and oxidative stress ensues, ROS may cause damage to various biological molecules and cellular components such as DNA, proteins, carbohydrates, lipids that are very sensitive to oxidation, and membranes [8,14].

Similarly, increased production of reactive nitrogen species (RNS) is termed a nitrosative stress. Nitric oxide (NO), the most potent vascular relaxing factor and a free radical, is an important mediator of the cardio- and cerebrovascular system. Nitric oxide is synthesized from arginine and O_2 by NO synthase (NOS). There are three NOS isozymes: neuronal (nNOS or NOS-1), cytokine-inducible in leukocytes (iNOS or NOS-2), and endothelial (eNOS or NOS-3) [15]. Nitric oxide is essential for vascular integrity, cardiovascular function, cerebral blood flow, cerebral vasodilation, and autoregulation. However, in a state of increased oxidative stress, NO levers are diminished via its interaction with superoxide anions yielding the potent radical peroxynitrite ($ONOO^-$) [16].

Ischemia/reperfusion is another well-established pathway of excessive ROS production. Oxygen desaturation as a result of apneas/hypopneas in patients with OSA is followed intermittently by a rapid reoxygenation of the blood-activating enzymes such as xanthine oxidase and NADPH oxidase. This phenomenon of hypoxia/reoxygenation, the hallmark of OSA, could be considered analogous to ischemia/reperfusion injury, thus leading to increased oxidative stress [14]. Reperfusion injury caused by a massive oxygenated blood flow following removal of blockage or return of cardiac function can aggravate the outcome of cerebral ischemia by increased ROS production. Thus, one of the major outcomes of stroke is ischemia/reperfusion injury to the central nervous system (CNS). Central nervous system ischemia/reperfusion injury is characterized by disruption of the blood–brain barrier, transmigration of leukocytes into the brain tissue, and increased ROS production by leukocytes as well, which can irreversibly damage surrounding cells including neurons [17].

Reactive oxygen species production and oxidative stress in obstructive sleep apnea and in animal models of intermittent hypoxia

Most studies investigating oxidative stress in patients with OSA present indirect findings by using various bodily fluid markers such as plasma, serum, or urine. Thiobarbituric acid-reactive substances (TBARS) and peroxides that represent by-products of lipid peroxidation are the most widely used. Figures 2.1A and B depict the differences in these markers between age-, gender-, and BMI-matched OSA and controls. Moreover, TBARS were strongly correlated with the apnea/hypopnea index in non-obese patients and matched controls (Figure 2.1C) [18]. Elevated plasma and exhaled levels of 8-isoprostane were also shown in patients with OSA [19,20]. Increased oxidative stress in OSA was shown by diminution in plasma total antioxidant activity and trolox equivalent antioxidant assay as well as small antioxidant molecules such as vitamin A, vitamin E, and gamma-glutamyltransferase levels. In addition, the activity of paraoxinase-1 (PON1), which is an antioxidant enzyme located exclusively on high density lipoprotein (HDL) and protects both HDL and low density lipoprotein (LDL) from oxidative modification, was shown to decrease in OSA (Figure 2.1D) [18].

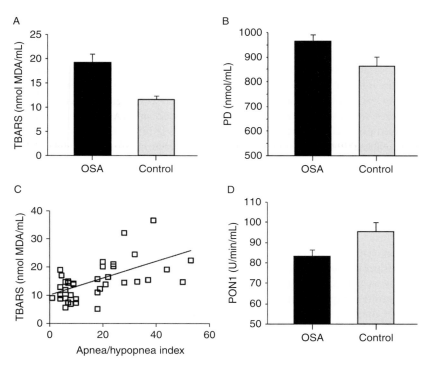

Figure 2.1. Oxidative stress markers in non-obese matched obstructive sleep apnea (OSA) patients (N=20) and controls (N=20). (A): thiobarbituric-acid-reactive substances (TBARS), P<0.0002; (B): peroxides (PD), P<0.03; (C): correlation between TBARS and the severity of OSA by apnea/hypopnea index (r=0.57, P<0.002); (D): paraoxonase-1 (PON1) levels, P<0.02. Values represent mean (± SEM). (Adapted from Lavie et al. [18]).

Treatment of OSA patients with nCPAP attenuated TBARS and peroxides [14,21] as well as exhaled isoprostanes levels [20]. More recently, Oyama et al. [22] confirmed previous studies reporting that nCPAP therapy significantly decreased the levels of markers associated with oxidative stress as decreased TBARS, increased NO levels, and decreased asymmetrical dimethylarginine. Additionally, nCPAP therapy was shown to improve the total antioxidant status and gamma-glutamyltransferase activity [23].

However, thus far only a few studies have demonstrated direct evidence for ROS production in OSA patients. Phagocytic cells release enormous amounts of ROS via activation of NADPH oxidase when encountering inflammatory/infectious microorganisms. However, activation by various stimuli including intermittent hypoxia (IH) also activates leukocyte NADPH oxidase. Schulz et al. have shown that OSA neutrophils stimulated by the microbial peptide FMLP (formylmethionyl-leucyl-phenylalanine) generated higher amounts of NADPH-dependent ROS than neutrophils obtained from controls [24]. Dyugovskaya et al. [25] have also shown that monocytes and granulocytes of OSA patients generated higher amounts of NADPH oxidase-dependent ROS than controls in response to phorbol myristate acetate (PMA). More importantly, monocytes were shown to produce higher amounts of ROS in OSA, also in the basal state, without additional stimulation, while treatment with nCPAP attenuated leukocyte ROS formation in both studies.

The NADPH oxidase isoforms are expressed in a variety of other cells. In the vasculature they generate ROS at lower rates for signaling purposes. Of note, apart from OSA, endothelial NADPH oxidase is also activated by IH. Increased ROS generation in the vascular wall of patients with OSA can lead to the development of inflammatory diseases including atherosclerosis, diabetes, and hypertension. Furthermore, a recent study by Pierola et al. [19] reported that the distribution of NADPH oxidase allelic polymorphs differed between OSA and controls. The risk of OSA was independently associated with A-930G polymorphisms of the p22phox gene, which was associated with the development of oxidative stress in these patients. Gozal et al. [26] have also shown that NADPH oxidase activity was higher in children with OSA and was associated with polymorphisms within the NADPH oxidase gene or its functional subunits and with cognitive functional deficits.

The importance of NADPH oxidase was shown in a number of murine models of IH mimicking OSA. For instance, oxidative stress responses and neurobehavioral impairments were mediated by increased NADPH oxidase activity [27]. Interestingly, exposure of mice to sleep fragmentation, which is an important component of OSA, significantly increased NADPH oxidase gene expression and activity, as well as markers of oxidative stress such as malondialdehyde and 8-oxo-2'-deoxyguanosine in cortical and hippocampal lysates [28].

Increased levels of xanthine oxidase were also reported in patients with OSA [29]. High levels of fatty acids in the brain make it a very susceptible tissue for lipid peroxidation. Thus, elevated levels of xanthine oxidase in patients with OSA can lead to lipid peroxidation and protein degradation in brain tissue. Moreover, El Solh et al. [30] reported, in a randomized study, that allopurinol, the potent xanthine oxidase inhibitor, significantly reduced lipid peroxidation and improved endothelial function in patients with moderate to severe OSA. In a recent study conducted on rats, xanthine oxidase was shown to play a key role in mediating intermittent hypoxia-induced vascular dysfunction in skeletal muscle resistance arteries [31]. Additionally, nitrosative stress was documented in OSA. Jelic et al. [32] reported that endothelial nitrotyrosine was five-fold higher in patients with OSA than in control subjects and was significantly decreased after nCPAP therapy.

Collectively, an enormous amount of direct and indirect data demonstrate elevated levels of oxidative/nitrosative stress markers in OSA, which can be attenuated by efficient nCPAP therapy. These findings were further corroborated by animal models of IH.

Oxidative stress in cardiovascular morbidity and stroke

As mentioned earlier, in acute ischemic stroke or myocardial infarction blood flow to the affected tissue is insufficient. Postischemic reperfusion may induce excessive ROS formation and contribute to tissue damage. Indeed, increased production of free radicals and subsequent oxidative stress were shown to affect the pathogenesis of stroke and may worsen the clinical outcome. Senes et al. [16] reported that acute ischemic stroke patients exhibit abnormalities in oxidative and nitrosative stress markers. Nitrite and nitrate, ischemia-modified albumin (IMA), and TBARS were significantly increased in stroke patients within the first 24 h from the onset of symptoms, as compared to age- and gender-matched controls. Furthermore, ischemia-induced ROS generation affects neuronal injury through several mechanisms including N-methyl-D-aspartate (NMDA) receptors, mitochondrial dysfunction, activation and induction of neuronal NOS (NOS-1) and cyclo-oxigenase 2, autooxidation of catecholamines, metabolism of free fatty acids, and leukocyte migration and activation [33]. Because brain tissues are extremely susceptible to oxidative/nitrosative stress injury, the increased production of free radicals resulting from the IH in patients with OSA may lead to neuronal damage and exacerbate clinical outcomes after stroke.

Vascular inflammation

Vascular inflammation is a multifactorial pathophysiological process, which is associated with a great number of diseases including coronary artery disease, atherosclerosis, and stroke as well as sleep apnea. In her seminal paper, Lavie [14] suggested that IH in patients with OSA during sleep can initiate complex metabolic molecular and cellular changes and promote development of vascular inflammation, leading to atherosclerosis. Elevated markers of vascular inflammation, such as oxidized LDL, C-reactive protein, markers of hypercoagulability and the fibrinolytic system, adhesion molecules, proinflammatory cytokines, and transcription factors have all been shown to be altered in patients with OSA. Moreover, inflammatory cell activation in leukocytes and platelets were described as well. Jointly, a proinflammatory and a prothrombotic phenotype is evident in OSA. The significance of vascular inflammation and some of the markers associated with it in stroke patients with OSA will be discussed in this section.

Oxidized low density lipoprotein

One of the most established markers of early atherosclerosis is the uptake of lipoproteins by monocytes/macrophages into subendothelial spaces. Lipoproteins are the major lipid carriers in the circulation. There are five major types of lipoproteins in the blood termed according to increasing density. Low density lipoprotein is the main cholesterol carrier in the plasma. In its native form, LDL does not induce cholesterol accumulation within the endothelial wall. However, high ROS levels can lead to LDL cholesterol oxidation and formation of oxidized LDL (oxLDL), which promotes pathological processes through uncontrolled oxLDL uptake and foam cell formation. Aggregation of oxLDL in the subendothelial layer of the arteries affects endothelial, smooth muscle, and inflammatory cell functions. Oxidized LDL can also induce apoptosis of vascular endothelial cells and lead to plaque formation and rupture. Oxidized LDL is also a potent inducer of mitochondrial ROS production, leading to caspase activation and apoptosis [34], as well as diminution of intracellular NO concentrations in endothelial cells [35]. Besides its crucial role in the pathogenesis of atherosclerosis through cholesterol deposition in the vessel wall, oxLDL can induce immune responses, which promote vascular inflammation and consequently atherosclerosis [36].

The presence of high oxLDL levels was shown in atherosclerotic lesions in humans as well as in animal models of atherosclerosis [37]. Moreover, it was shown to induce atherogenesis by several mechanisms including recruitment of circulating monocytes into the intimal space, induction of macrophage survival [38], foam cell formation, and disruption of endothelial integrity. In addition, oxLDL activates endothelial cells and platelet aggregation [36].

Increased circulating levels of oxLDL were reported in a number of studies investigating patients with OSA. Additionally, autoantibodies against oxLDL were shown to increase as compared to controls. Barceló et al. [39] have shown that the level of oxidation of LDL was increased in patients with OSA and their LDL was more susceptible to oxidation than that in controls. These measures were improved by nCPAP treatment [39]. In addition, increased oxLDL-mediated lectin-like oxidized LDL receptor-1 (LOX-1) upregulation was associated with endothelial injury in OSA patients [40]. Increased LOX-1 expression in OSA was associated with endothelial cell apoptosis and was decreased by nCPAP therapy [41]. Patients with OSA also expressed a degree of HDL dysfunction and concomitant increase in oxLDL levels [42]. It was suggested that dysfunctional HDL, which has antiatherogenic and antioxidant properties, may contribute to increased cerebrovascular risk in patients with OSA [42]. In a recent American Thoracic Society symposium, Mehra et al. [43] reported that, in a large cohort of patients with sleep-disordered breathing, an increased oxidized LDL/total LDL ratio was associated with nocturnal hypoxia but not with an AHI, suggesting that the hypoxia burden rather than the frequency of respiratory events was a risk factor for increased lipid peroxidation.

Elevated oxLDL levels were also reported in patients with cardiovascular morbidity including stable angina, unstable angina, and acute myocardial infarction. Because oxLDL participates in the initiation and progression of atherosclerosis and is involved in foam cell formation and late-stage plaque instability and rupture, the association between oxLDL and stroke was investigated. Compared to controls, oxLDL levels were markedly higher in acute stroke patients [44,45]. In addition, a persistent increase in plasma oxLDL was associated with enlargement of the ischemic lesion in the early phase after the insult [46]. Moreover, in a cross-sectional population-based study of 513 men, all 61 years old, oxLDL was independently associated with the occurrence of echolucent plaques in the carotid artery [47]. These findings suggest that oxLDL plays a central role in the pathogenesis of stroke and recovery. Thus, increased oxLDL levels associated with OSA may further exacerbate its effects on cardio- and cerebrovascular morbidity associated with OSA.

High sensitivity C-reactive protein

High sensitivity C-reactive protein (hsCRP) is one of the most highly investigated mediators of vascular inflammation and atherosclerosis. Increased hsCRP levels were identified as a risk factor for the development of ischemic heart disease and ischemic cerebrovascular disease. Furthermore, hsCRP was documented in many epidemiological studies as a strong predictor of coronary heart disease and of future cardiovascular events [8]. High sensitivity CRP is

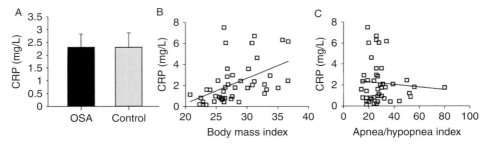

Figure 2.2. (A): C-reactive protein (CRP) in non-obese patients with obstructive sleep apnea (OSA) (N=20) and individually matched controls (N=20) (NS); (B): correlation between CRP and body mass index (BMI) in patients with OSA (r=0.49, P<0.0001); (C): correlation between CRP and the severity of OSA measured by the apnea/hypopnea index (r=-0.08, NS). In (B) and (C), 46 non-obese and obese OSA patients were included. NS, not significant. (Adapted from Lavie et al. [18]).

produced primarily by the liver in response to inflammatory cytokines such as interleukin-6 (IL-6) and tumor necrosis factor-alpha (TNF-α), but it is also produced by nonhepatic tissues. In addition, hsCRP can accelerate atherogenic processes by initiating endothelial dysfunction via induction of adhesion molecules and inhibition of NO-mediated dilation in the vasculature by inhibiting endothelial NOS.

Studies reported to date on circulating hsCRP levels in patients with OSA are inconsistent. The first study by Shamsuzzaman et al. [48] demonstrated that hsCRP was increased in obese OSA in a severity-dependent manner. Similar findings were reported by Yokoe et al. [49] in obese patients and controls, while one month of nCPAP treatment dramatically decreased hsCRP levels. This was further demonstrated after three and six months of treatment [50]. In additional studies, obesity rather than sleep apnea was suggested as a risk factor for increased hsCRP levels in OSA [51]. Lavie et al. [18] did not find differences in hsCRP levels between non-obese patients and controls matched by age and gender (Figure 2.2A). However, hsCRP levels were shown to be BMI- rather than AHI dependent in otherwise matched patients groups, which differed only in BMI (Figures 2.2B and C). A recent study confirmed that hsCRP levels were primarily associated with BMI and less so with the AHI. However, in multiple regression analysis, elevated hsCRP levels were associated with the AHI independent of obesity [52]. Gender specificity was also reported to affect hsCRP levels after nCPAP treatment; in males hsCRP levels were decreased by three months of treatment, while in females hsCRP levels were decreased only after six months [50]. Sleep deprivation can also induce hsCRP elevation. It is thus difficult to separate the independent contribution of each of the variables affecting hsCRP in OSA [53]. However, pathological hsCRP levels ($\geq$3 mg/L) were more prevalent in patients with severe OSA [54]. Elevated hsCRP levels were also reported on comorbidity-free middle-aged men with OSA in association with severity and independent of visceral obesity. After adjusting for age, smoking, BMI, waist circumference, and sleep efficiency, hsCRP was positively correlated with the AHI, duration of O_2 saturation of <90%, and arousal index [55]. In addition, in patients with severe OSA with significantly higher hsCRP levels, heart rate recovery at 1 min after exercise termination (HRR-1), peak heart rate, and peak of oxygen consumption (VO(2peak)) values were lower than those of controls. The hsCRP levels correlated significantly with impaired HRR-1 in the OSA group after adjustment for VO(2peak) [56]. Consequently, good nCPAP compliance followed for one year resulted in a significant hsCRP reduction and had a positive impact on cardiovascular morbidity and mortality [57].

In a large cross-sectional study in the United States, hsCRP concentration was higher in patients with than without stroke, therefore suggesting that hsCRP levels may be a risk factor or a marker of stroke [58]. Moreover, hsCRP levels were shown to be an independent predictor of survival after an ischemic stroke [59]. Furthermore, in stroke patients with OSA, hsCRP levels were higher as compared to stroke patients without OSA [60], and were found to predict the severity of OSA apnea in stroke patients [61]. It was thus suggested that high hsCRP levels in patients with OSA may worsen the recovery and increase the risk for mortality after stroke regardless of whether hsCRP levels are increased because of apnea severity, obesity, or stroke. Therefore, routine determination of hsCRP levels should be considered in patients with OSA and in obese OSA in particular.

Hypercoagulability and fibrinolysis

Impaired fibrinolytic activity and hypercoagulability are implicated in the development of the majority of acute cerebrocardiovascular events such as stroke and myocardial infarction. Increased coagulation and decreased fibrinolytic activity are highly prevalent among OSA patients as well [62]. Fibrinogen is the major procoagulant molecule, whereas plasminogen activator inhibitor-1 (PAI-1) is a pivotal mediator of the fibrinolytic system [4,62]. Elevated levels of fibrinogen and/or PAI-1 can lead to an imbalance in the fibrinolytic system and predispose OSA patients to stroke.

Elevated PAI-1 levels were reported in patients with OSA and were correlated with OSA severity [4]. In endothelial cells, elevated PAI-1 expression was associated with impaired endothelial function. Several physiological and pathophysiological stimuli were shown to induce PAI-1 expression in endothelial cells. Among others, hypoxia, ROS, and angiotensin II (Ang II) are the most potent activators of PAI-1 gene expression [4,63]. The presence of such activators in patients with OSA increases PAI-1 levels and affects the fibrinolytic activity, and may lead to the development of stroke. In addition, Ang II is a potent vaso-constrictor peptide. Thus, high Ang II levels in patients with OSA [40] can cause sympathetic activation, leading to hypertension [64], a well-known risk factor for stroke.

Fibrinogen is a procoagulant plasma protein. It is synthesized in the liver and is upregulated in response to several physiological and pathophysiological phenomena, such as infection or inflammation, wound healing, tumorigenesis, and atherosclerosis. It is an important hemo-static mediator in blood coagulation, blood rheology, and platelet aggregation. Fibrinogen may directly damage the vascular wall through endothelial cell injury or by stimulating smooth muscle proliferation and migration [65]. Thus, elevated plasma fibrinogen levels are an important independent risk factor for cardiocerebrovascular events such as myocardial infarction and stroke [66]. Moreover, high plasma fibrinogen levels were shown to be an independent risk factor for cardiovascular events in patients who survived stroke. In the Northwick Park Heart study, an increase in fibrinogen concentration was associated with an 84% increase in the risk of ischemic heart disease within the following five years. Furthermore, in OSA, effective nCPAP treatment reduced morning plasma fibrinogen levels and whole blood viscosity [67]. In addition, in patients with OSA and stroke, plasma fibrinogen levels were positively correlated with the AHI and negatively with minimal and average minimal oxygen saturation [67]. Based on these findings, fibrinogen might be considered as a possible pathophysiological link between sleep apnea and stroke. A higher risk of stroke recurrence and other vascular events, including myocardial infarction in stroke patients with OSA, signify the importance of the treatment of OSA [11].

Nuclear factor-kappaB and hypoxia-inducible factor-1α transcription factors

Data from sleep apnea patients as well as from animal models of IH showed that inflammatory responses resulting from a hypoxia/reoxygenation insult can stimulate a number of redox-sensitive transcription factors. Two of the most important redox-regulated transcription factors are hypoxia-inducible factor-1α (HIF-1α) and nuclear factor-kappaB (NF-κB).

The factor NF-κB is a master regulator of inflammatory gene expression. Activation of the NF-κB pathway can lead to expression of a variety of factors, including cytokines (TNF-α, IL-6, and IL-8), adhesion molecules (intercellular adhesion molecule-1), and enzymes (cyclooxygenase-2) [8]. Higher activity of NF-κB was reported in monocytes and neutrophils of OSA patients, whereas treatment with nCPAP significantly decreased its activation [68,69]. Moreover, exposure of human polymorphonuclear cells (PMNs) to IH in vitro stimulated NF-κB nuclear translocation [68,70]. Thus, expression of downstream inflammatory cytokines and adhesion molecules in OSA likely results from NF-κB activation.

The factor HIF-1α is a master regulator of adaptive responses to hypoxia through the expression of hundreds of genes, such as vascular endothelial growth factor (VEGF), erythropoietin (EPO), as well as proinflammatory cytokines and chemokines. Vascular endothelial growth factor is one of the most important downstream genes regulated by HIF-1α to counteract ischemic/hypoxic conditions [71]; it is a potent vasodilator and angiogenic factor in normal physiological and pathophysiological conditions. It also promotes the expression of vascular cell adhesion molecule 1 (VCAM-1) and intercellular adhesion molecule 1 (ICAM-1) in endothelial cells. In addition, VEGF can activate tissue-type plasminogen activators (t-PA) and PAI-1 expression in cultured microvascular endothelial cells [72]. Vascular endothelial growth factor is also vital for recruiting endothelial progenitor cells (EPCs) to the circulation and promotes the development of coronary collateral arteries. As a result, VEGF can protect the myocardium from severe ischemic injury [73]. Altogether, VEGF plays a major compensating role in hypoxia and ischemia/reperfusion conditions.

In patients with OSA, circulating VEGF levels were shown to increase in a severity-dependent manner and were decreased by nCPAP therapy [73]. Similarly, VEGF levels were increased in stroke patients and were correlated with the severity of stroke, indicating that VEGF may play an important role in the pathophysiology of acute ischemic stroke [74]. Angiogenesis, which is mediated mainly by VEGF, is essential for the recovery of ischemic brain tissue. Stroke patients with a high density of cerebral blood vessels are likely to survive longer than patients with low vascular density. Furthermore, in animal brains exposed to ischemia, increased cerebral angiogenesis by cell-based and pharmacological therapies was associated with improvement in functional outcome and recovery [75].

Erythropoietin (EPO), another downstream gene product of HIF-1α and a major mediator of erythropoiesis, was also investigated in OSA. Winnicki et al. [76] reported that patients with severe OSA had significantly increased EPO levels, which were decreased after nCPAP treatment. Moreover, increased erythrocyte adhesiveness and aggregation was shown in patients with OSA as compared to controls [77]. Elevated EPO levels and increased erythrocyte aggregation/adhesion may also contribute to the higher rates of cardiovascular morbidity in OSA.

Although HIF-1α mediates mostly adaptive responses to hypoxia, it also enhances the survival of myeloid inflammatory cells, such as granulocytes, monocytes, and macrophages, leading to their functional longevity and exacerbation of inflammation. Furthermore, a cross-talk between NF-κB and HIF-1α pathways was suggested to modulate the inflammatory response to intermittent hypoxia in OSA [78]. Walmsley et al. [79] showed that the presence of HIF-1α is required for the hypoxic induction of NF-κB transcription and that hypoxia-induced neutrophil survival was regulated by HIF-1α through the NF-κB signaling pathway. It is a likely possibility that the HIF-1α pathway is activated in patients with severe OSA as downstream genes like VEGF and EPO are upregulated in OSA [14]. However, HIF-1α activation was demonstrated only in animal models of IH [80].

Proinflammatory cytokines

Proinflammatory cytokines are increased in patients with OSA as well as in patients with stroke and cerebral ischemia. Recurrent episodes of hypoxia/reoxygenation in patients with sleep apnea and stroke may lead to increased levels of the inflammatory cytokines in the brain and worsen the clinical outcome after stroke.

Tumor necrosis factor-α is a central cytokine with pleiotropic proinflammatory activity in atherosclerotic processes. It is primarily synthesized by macrophages, but is also produced by a wide range of cell types including lymphoid cells, mast cells, endothelial cells, cardiac myocytes, adipose tissue, fibroblasts, and neuronal tissue.

Tumor necrosis factor-α is one of the most studied cytokines in OSA. Although the findings regarding circulating TNF-α levels are somewhat inconsistent, most studies have shown increases in the levels of circulating TNF-α in patients with OSA [81]. Moreover, these increases were independent of central obesity [82]. Additionally, in monocytes of patients with moderate to severe OSA, spontaneous TNF-α production was increased [83]. Similarly, spontaneous TNF-α production was increased in the cytotoxic T lymphocytes of patients with OSA [84]. Interestingly, the levels of soluble TNF receptor-1 (sTNFR-1) were shown to increase significantly in OSA as compared with controls [85]. High TNF-α levels can lead to increased ROS production and upregulation of adhesion molecules. Moreover, TNF-α can stimulate the synthesis of other cytokines, such as IL-6, through the NF-κB transcriptional pathway. Interleukin-6 is secreted by T cells and macrophages and promotes immune responses, leading to inflammation. In addition, IL-6 is an atherogenic marker associated with the development of coronary heart disease and a predictor of cardiovascular risk beyond traditional risk factors in aged populations [86]. Increased levels of TNF-α and IL-6 in patients with OSA were significantly decreased with nCPAP therapy [22].

In stroke patients, TNF-α levels were increased in the cerebrospinal fluid and in sera in the first 24 h of the onset of symptoms [87]. Tumor necrosis factor-α was shown to stimulate the synthesis of IL-6 and promote inflammatory responses after stroke. In addition, in stroke patients who were diagnosed with OSA, IL-6 was significantly increased in the first week after the stroke. Among cases with acute stroke and severe OSA, IL-6 levels were correlated with lower oxyhemoglobin desaturation and with the desaturation index [9]. These finding suggest that IL-6 might be associated with the development of atherogenesis in OSA patients with cerebrovascular disease.

Interleukin-10 (IL-10) is another cytokine with potential implications for OSA. Unlike TNF-α or IL-6, it is an antiinflammatory and antiatherogenic cytokine. It is secreted by a wide range of immune cells including monocytes, mast cells, and also in a certain subset of activated T, B, and NK cells. Interleukin-10 attenuates the production of proinflammatory cytokines, including TNF-α, suppresses antigen-presenting activity, attenuates ROS production, and affects adhesion of monocytes and endothelial cells. Circulating levels of IL-10 were shown to decrease significantly in patients with OSA compared to matched controls [81]. Vila et al. [88] showed (using the Canadian Stroke Scale) that IL-10 levels were significantly decreased in stroke patients with neurological worsening within the first 48 h after admission. These findings indicate that IL-10 might be associated with early stages of clinical recovery after acute ischemic stroke.

Interleukin-12 (IL-12) is another proinflammatory cytokine with potential implications for OSA by virtue of its active role during the early phase of atherosclerosis. Interleukin-12 was shown to increase the production of TNF-α, while IL-10 downregulates IL-12 production and proinflammatory cytokine responses. Interestingly, LDL induces IL-10 production, whereas oxLDL induces IL-12 production from macrophages [89]. In OSA, nasal lavage levels of IL-12 were attenuated after nCPAP treatment combined with heated humidification, as compared to sham-heated humidification [90], indicating that its levels might be increased in OSA. Additionally, the levels of IL-12 were shown to increase in acute stroke patients within 24–72 hours from onset of the symptoms compared to matched controls [91,92]. Moreover, IL-12 levels were correlated with the Scandinavian Score Scale and erythrocyte sedimentation values. Therefore, it was suggested that IL-12 might be implicated in the pathophysiology of ischemic stroke.

Adhesion molecules

Adhesion molecules are glycoproteins expressed on the cell surface of leukocytes and endothelial cells. They are upregulated in response to a variety of stimuli, including hypoxia/reoxygenation and OSA. Adhesion molecules promote cellular interactions between various leukocyte subpopulations, platelets, and endothelial cells. The adhesion cascade of leukocytes to endothelial cells involves multiple independent steps, including rolling, firm adhesion, and transmigration [93]. The family of selectins (L-, E-, and P-) regulate leukocyte rolling on the endothelium. The firm adhesion involves interaction between β2-integrins (mainly of the CD11a/CD18 and CD11b/CD18) on leukocytes with ICAM-1 and VCAM-1 on endothelial cells. The firm adhesion is followed by transmigration of the leukocytes across the endothelium to target tissues, where they release ROS, proinflammatory cytokines, and proteolytic enzymes [94].

In OSA, leukocyte activation and upregulation of the adhesion molecules has been reported in monocytes and lymphocytes [95]. Adhesion molecules in the circulation derived from endothelial cells were also increased in OSA, while elevated ICAM-1, VCAM-1, L-selectin, and E-selectin levels were attenuated by nCPAP treatment [96]. Jointly, these observations suggest that the endothelium and leukocytes of patients with OSA are activated and that treatment with nCPAP can ameliorate this condition. Circulating levels of soluble ICAM-1, VCAM-1, and E-selectin were significantly increased in OSA patients with coronary artery disease compared to matched controls without OSA [97]. These findings suggest that OSA can modulate the expression of adhesion molecules regardless of a potential contribution of confounders such as coronary artery disease and left ventricular dysfunction [29]. Furthermore, E-selectin was reported as an independent proatherogenic factor in patients with OSA [98]. In vitro activation and aggregation of platelets are increased in OSA. The percentage of platelets expressing P-selectin (CD62P) is higher, particularly in patients with severe OSA, and is lowered effectively after nCPAP treatment [99]. Collectively, elevated levels of ICAM-1, VCAM-1, E-selectin, and P-selectin further imply that OSA is a predisposing factor for atherogenesis.

In stroke, brain ischemia, which activates the cerebral microvascular endothelium, is accompanied by upregulation of adhesion molecules promoting the recruitment of leukocytes and platelets. Excessive accumulation of inflammatory cells in the ischemic area may further damage the brain tissue by releasing ROS and other inflammatory mediators. Thus, brain tissue injury in stroke patients, resulting in leukocyte infiltration and activation, can be exaggerated by the IH in patients with OSA and stroke. Moreover, it has been suggested that firm binding of platelets to adherent leukocytes may further activate both cell types and exacerbate tissue injury [100]. Jointly, these data indicate that increased expression of adhesion molecules in stroke patients with OSA may promote brain injury and worsen the clinical outcome after stroke.

Endothelial dysfunction

The endothelium is a dynamic tissue/monolayer lining the inner surface of blood vessels. It regulates vascular tone, structure, and inflammation by releasing vasodilative and vasoconstrictive mediators. In addition, the endothelium provides protective functions and a structural barrier between the circulatory system and the tissues. Nitric oxide is the most important vasodilator. Under normal conditions, endothelial cells constitutively express endothelial NOS (eNOS); it can be induced further by several physiological and pathophysiological extracellular stimuli such as insulin, shear stress, and cytokines [101].

Exposure to oxidative stress and proinflammatory mediators is frequently associated with activation of endothelial cells, leading to impaired endothelial function. This condition is defined as endothelial dysfunction and refers to a loss of normal homeostatic functions in blood vessels. A large body of evidence demonstrates that endothelial dysfunction is a frequent consequence of OSA, leading to alterations in vascular functions and structures, reduced endothelial repair capacity, and vascular reactivity. Endothelial dysfunction is also associated with increased platelet adhesion and aggregation, leukocyte/endothelial adhesion, and smooth muscle cell proliferation. High ROS levels, which neutralize NO and its antiatherogenic properties, initiate the development of vascular plaques, linking endothelial dysfunction to atherosclerosis [102]. Indeed, diminished NO bioavailability in patients with OSA has been previously reported by several studies [103]. Collectively, these inflammatory consequences can exacerbate vascular damage, establishing OSA as an independent risk factor for endothelial dysfunction [104].

Itzhaki et al. [105] reported that morning index of endothelial function was significantly lower in patients with moderate to severe OSA than in patients with mild sleep apnea or in the control group. Endothelial dysfunction was associated with increased oxidative stress in mild to moderate OSA. Treatment with the Herbst mandibular advancement splint decreased the AHI and improved endothelial function as well as oxidative stress markers [106]. In addition, Oyama et al. [22] demonstrated in a recent study that the AHI was correlated with endothelial function, measured by the forearm blood flow response to reactive hyperemia, which was significantly increased after three months of CPAP applications. Jelic et al. [107] showed that OSA alone impaired endothelial repair capacity and promoted endothelial apoptosis in non-obese, comorbidity-free patients. Baseline flow-mediated dilation was lower in patients with OSA compared to controls and was significantly increased by effective nCPAP treatment [32].

Endothelial dysfunction was suggested as a potential mechanism for stroke pathophysiology, clinical severity, and outcome. Freestone et al. [108] reported that endothelial dysfunction, as measured by decreased flow-mediated dilation, increased the risk of stroke in patients with atrial fibrillation. Thus, impaired endothelial function, particularly in patients with severe OSA, may promote the development of atherogenic processes and stroke.

The role of endothelial progenitor cells (EPCs) in endothelial function

There has been growing evidence in recent years that NO is a powerful mediator of new vessel formation and angiogenesis. Moreover, NO was shown to regulate protective functions of the endothelium such as recruitment of EPCs. Endothelial progenitor cells are bone marrow-derived pluripotent cells that participate in restoration of damaged blood vessels, particularly after an ischemic injury.

To date, findings on EPC levels in OSA are still an ongoing debate. In several studies, decreased numbers of circulating EPCs in comorbidity-free patients with OSA have been reported, whereas in other studies no differences in EPC levels were found [73]. In addition, nCPAP treatment was shown to increase EPC recruitment and improved vascular function in OSA patients with endothelial dysfunction [107]. Furthermore, EPC levels were negatively correlated with impaired endothelial function in children with OSA [109]. A recent study by Butt et al. [110] reported that EPC levels did not differ between patients with OSA and controls. It was indicated that EPCs were not associated with endothelial dysfunction in myocardial perfusion in patients with moderate to severe OSA. We have recently completed a study on patients with acute myocardial infarction (AMI) with and without SDB. We found that coexistent SDB in AMI patients significantly increased EPC mobilization, function, and angiogenic properties. Intermittent hypoxia in vitro significantly increased the function and angiogenic properties of EPCs from healthy individuals, indicating that IH associated with SDB is a major contributor to EPC recruitment and activation (Beger et al. unpublished observations). Jointly, these contrasting findings indicate that not all patients with OSA are susceptible to the negative consequences of hypoxia/reoxygenation to the same degree. Moreover, it is likely that IH may activate adaptive mechanisms and confer protection by recruitment of progenitor cells to the cardiocerebrovascular system.

Data on EPC levels in patients with stroke are very limited. However, it was suggested that EPCs may play a role in the pathophysiology of cerebrovascular disease and contribute to the maintenance of the cerebral circulation in postischemic injury [111]. Evidence from animal models of stroke demonstrated that higher EPC numbers and functions were associated with neurovascular repair, and improved long-term neurobehavioral outcomes [112]. Thus, the link between angiogenesis and neurogenesis in the poststroke brain and ongoing clinical trials on cell-based therapies for patients with stroke show great promise. However, additional studies are required to determine the therapeutic potential of EPCs in stroke.

Atherosclerosis in sleep apnea

Atherosclerosis is a progressive disease characterized by the accumulation of lipids and fibrous elements in the large arteries. Atherosclerosis is now considered as a chronic inflammatory response, implicating activated endothelium, leukocytes, platelets, and intimal smooth muscle cells. Epidemiological studies over the last 40–50 years identified a great number of risk factors for atherosclerosis. Among them are age, gender, obesity, cigarette smoking, hypertension, diabetes mellitus, plasma homocysteine, and serum cholesterol.

In the last decade, OSA has also been implicated as one of the risk factors inducing atherosclerosis [113]. Several cross-sectional studies have shown consistently that OSA is independently associated with surrogate markers of premature atherosclerosis. For instance,

Suzuki et al. [114] reported that the severity of OSA was independently related to atherogenic thickening of the carotid artery wall as measured by ultrasonic evaluation of intima–media thickness (IMT). Baguet et al. [115] reported that the severity of oxygen desaturation predicted carotid IMT and plaque occurrence in OSA patients without known cardiovascular disease. Using ultrasound imaging, the coronary atherosclerotic volume was shown to be greater in patients with an AHI of >15 compared to patients with an AHI of <15 events/h. Moreover, the coronary atherosclerotic plaque volume was significantly positively correlated with the AHI [116]. Importantly, Drager et al. [117] reported that nCPAP treatment significantly improved early signs of atherosclerosis, such as IMT and pulse-wave velocity. In a randomized clinical trial, OSA treatment with nCPAP was shown to attenuate carotid artery atherosclerosis [118].

In stroke patients with OSA, a higher prevalence of internal carotid artery atherosclerotic lesions was found compared to that in stroke patients without OSA [119]. This finding emphasizes the potential contribution of OSA in increasing the risk for developing stroke through atherogenic pathways [11].

Protective mechanisms in sleep apnea

Although sleep apnea is a major independent risk factor for the development of stroke or acute myocardial infarction, not all OSA patients develop cerebrocardiovascular morbidity. In a great number of studies, ischemic preconditioning (IPC) was shown to protect the brain and heart from ischemic injury. Ischemic preconditioning is a general phenomenon characterized by repeated periods of sublethal ischemia, which can provide profound protection from ischemic insults. In addition, IPC was shown to protect various tissues such as skeletal muscles, gut, and liver from ischemic/hypoxic injury.

In sleep apnea, the repetitive episodes of IH may resemble the brief periods of ischemia/reperfusion and promote development of IPC in some patients. Ischemic preconditioning can induce recruitment and differentiation of bone marrow-derived progenitor cells and enhance postischemic tissue recovery. A preliminary report by Steiner et al. [120] demonstrated that OSA was associated with an increased development of coronary collateral vessels in patients with total coronary occlusion. Interestingly, although OSA is a well-known independent risk factor for the increased incidence of stroke and death, declining rates of mortality with age were observed in male patients with sleep apnea [121]. Lavie and Lavie [122] reported an unexpected survival advantage in elderly patients with moderate OSA in comparison with an age-, gender-, and ethnicity-matched cohort of the general population. Thus, based on these observations, it may be hypothesized that chronic IH might activate adaptive pathways that may confer cardioprotection in selected populations of patient populations with OSA [122,123] (see Figure 2.3.).

Conclusions

Obstructive sleep apnea is a multifactorial disorder, which is associated with the development of atherosclerosis and cardiocerebrovascular morbidity, including myocardial infarction and stroke. The presence of IH is a key factor in initiating proatherogenic activity and a likely link for the close association between OSA and cardiovascular diseases. Increased oxidative stress, vascular inflammation, and endothelial dysfunction resulting from IH can lead to high susceptibility of patients with OSA to stroke. On the other hand, IH may activate adaptive mechanisms, such as increased coronary heart collateralization and recruitment of

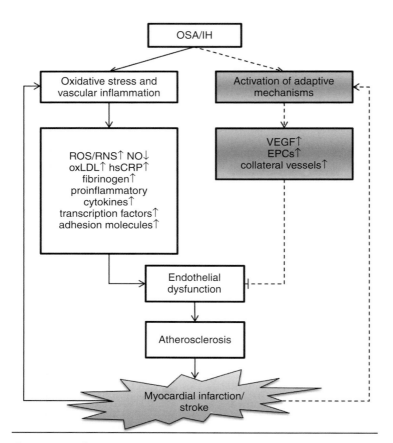

Figure 2.3. An illustration summarizing proatherogenic (solid lines) and possible adaptive pathways (dashed lines), affected by obstructive sleep apnea (OSA)/intermittent hypoxia (IH) and promoting or protecting from acute cardiocerebrovascular diseases. EPCs, endothelial progenitor cells; hsCRP, high sensitivity C-reactive protein; NO, nitric oxide; oxLDL, oxidized low density lipoprotein; RNS, reactive nitrogen species; ROS, reactive oxygen species; VEGF, vascular endothelial growth factor.

bone marrow-derived EPCs, which can provide protection to postischemic injured tissues. The balance between proatherogenic and protective mechanisms may determine the predisposition of OSA patients to stroke or other cardiocerebrovascular diseases. The findings described in this chapter and the course of events are illustrated in Figure 2.3.

References

1. McNicholas WT, Bonsigore MR, B26 MCoECA. Sleep apnoea as an independent risk factor for cardiovascular disease: current evidence, basic mechanisms and research priorities. *Eur Respir J* 2007; **29**: 156–78.

2. Punjabi NM. The epidemiology of adult obstructive sleep apnea. *Proc Am Thorac Soc* 2008; **5**: 136–43.

3. Cereda C, Lavie L, Bassetti CL. Sleep disordered breathing and stroke. In: Silvestri R, ed. *Sleep Disorders in Neurology*. New York, NY: Nova Science Publishers, 2012.

4. Bagai K. Obstructive sleep apnea, stroke, and cardiovascular diseases. *Neurologist* 2010; **16**: 329–39.

5. Young T, Palta M, Dempsey J, et al. The occurrence of sleep-disordered breathing among middle-aged adults. *N Engl J Med* 1993; **328**: 1230–5.

6. Milleron O, Pilliere R, Foucher A, et al. Benefits of obstructive sleep apnoea treatment in coronary artery disease: a long-term follow-up study. *Eur Heart J* 2004; **25**: 728–34.

7. Sobieszczyk P, Beckman J. Carotid artery disease. *Circulation* 2006; **114**: e244–7.

8. Lavie L, Lavie P. Molecular mechanisms of cardiovascular disease in OSAHS: the oxidative stress link. *Eur Respir J* 2009; **33**: 1467–84.

9. Medeiros CA, de Bruin VM, Andrade GM, et al. Obstructive sleep apnea and biomarkers of inflammation in ischemic stroke. *Acta Neurol Scand* 2012; **126**: 17–22.

10. Yaggi HK, Concato J, Kernan WN, et al. Obstructive sleep apnea as a risk factor for stroke and death. *N Engl J Med* 2005; **353**: 2034–41.

11. Redline S, Yenokyan G, Gottlieb DJ, et al. Obstructive sleep apnea-hypopnea and incident stroke: the Sleep Heart Health Study. *Am J Respir Crit Care Med* 2010; **182**: 269–77.

12. Martínez-García MA, Soler-Cataluña JJ, Ejarque-Martínez L, et al. Continuous positive airway pressure treatment reduces mortality in patients with ischemic stroke and obstructive sleep apnea: a 5-year follow-up study. *Am J Respir Crit Care Med* 2009; **180**: 36–41.

13. Martínez-García MA, Campos-Rodríguez F, Soler-Cataluña JJ, et al. Increased incidence of non-fatal cardiovascular events in stroke patients with sleep apnoea. Effect of CPAP treatment. *Eur Respir J* 2012; **39**: 906–12.

14. Lavie L. Obstructive sleep apnoea syndrome–an oxidative stress disorder. *Sleep Med Rev* 2003; **7**: 35–51.

15. Knowles RG, Moncada S. Nitric oxide synthases in mammals. *Biochem J*. 1994; **298**: 249–58.

16. Senes M, Kazan N, Coskun O, et al. Oxidative and nitrosative stress in acute ischaemic stroke. *Ann Clin Biochem* 2007; **44**: 43–7.

17. Saeed SA, Shad KF, Saleem T, et al. Some new prospects in the understanding of the molecular basis of the pathogenesis of stroke. *Exp Brain Res* 2007; **182**: 1–10.

18. Lavie L, Vishnevsky A, Lavie P. Oxidative stress and systemic inflammation in patients with sleep apnea: role of obesity. *Sleep Biol Rhythms* 2007; **5**: 100–10.

19. Pierola J, Alemany A, Yanez A, et al. NADPH oxidase p22phox polymorphisms and oxidative stress in patients with obstructive sleep apnoea. *Respir Med* 2011; **105**: 1748–54.

20. Carpagnano GE, Kharitonov SA, Resta O, et al. 8-Isoprostane, a marker of oxidative stress, is increased in exhaled breath condensate of patients with obstructive sleep apnea after night and is reduced by continuous positive airway pressure therapy. *Chest* 2003; **124**: 1386–92.

21. Lavie L, Vishnevsky A, Lavie P. Evidence for lipid peroxidation in obstructive sleep apnea. *Sleep* 2004; **27**: 123–8.

22. Oyama JI, Yamamoto H, Maeda T, et al. Continuous positive airway pressure therapy improves vascular dysfunction and decreases oxidative stress in patients with the metabolic syndrome and obstructive sleep apnea syndrome. *Clin Cardiol* 2012; **35**: 231–6.

23. Barceló A, Barbe F, de la Peña M, et al. Antioxidant status in patients with sleep apnoea and impact of continuous positive airway pressure treatment. *Eur Respir J* 2006; **27**: 756–60.

24. Schulz R, Mahmoudi S, Hattar K, et al. Enhanced release of superoxide from polymorphonuclear neutrophils in obstructive sleep apnea. Impact of continuous positive airway pressure therapy. *Am J Respir Crit Care Med* 2000; **162**: 566–70.

25. Dyugovskaya L, Lavie P, Lavie L. Increased adhesion molecules expression and production of reactive oxygen species in leukocytes of sleep apnea patients. *Am J Respir Crit Care Med* 2002; **165**: 934–9.

26. Gozal D, Khalyfa A, Capdevila OS, et al. Cognitive function in prepubertal children with obstructive sleep apnea: a modifying role for NADPH oxidase p22 subunit gene polymorphisms? *Antioxid Redox Signal* 2012; **16**: 171–7.

27. Nair D, Dayyat EA, Zhang SX, et al. Intermittent hypoxia-induced cognitive

deficits are mediated by NADPH oxidase activity in a murine model of sleep apnea. *PLoS One* 2011; **6**: e19847.

28. Nair D, Zhang SX, Ramesh V, et al. Sleep fragmentation induces cognitive deficits via NADPH oxidase-dependent pathways in mouse. *Am J Respir Crit Care Med* 2011; **184**: 1305–12.

29. Ramar K, Caples SM. Vascular changes, cardiovascular disease and obstructive sleep apnea. *Future Cardiol* 2011; **7**: 241–9.

30. El Solh AA, Saliba R, Bosinski T, et al. Allopurinol improves endothelial function in sleep apnoea: a randomised controlled study. *Eur Respir J* 2006; **27**: 997–1002.

31. Dopp JM, Philippi NR, Marcus NJ, et al. Xanthine oxidase inhibition attenuates endothelial dysfunction caused by chronic intermittent hypoxia in rats. *Respiration* 2011; **82**: 458–67.

32. Jelic S, Padeletti M, Kawut SM, et al. Inflammation, oxidative stress, and repair capacity of the vascular endothelium in obstructive sleep apnea. *Circulation* 2008; **117**: 2270–8.

33. Ozkul A, Akyol A, Yenisey C, et al. Oxidative stress in acute ischemic stroke. *J Clin Neurosci* 2007; **14**: 1062–6.

34. Littlewood TD, Bennett MR. Apoptotic cell death in atherosclerosis. *Curr Opin Lipidol* 2003; **14**: 469–75.

35. Cominacini L, Rigoni A, Pasini AF, et al. The binding of oxidized low density lipoprotein (ox-LDL) to ox-LDL receptor-1 reduces the intracellular concentration of nitric oxide in endothelial cells through an increased production of superoxide. *J Biol Chem* 2001; **276**: 13 750–5.

36. Grundtman C, Wick G. The autoimmune concept of atherosclerosis. *Curr Opin Lipidol* 2011; **22**: 327–34.

37. Mitra S, Goyal T, Mehta JL. Oxidized LDL, LOX-1 and atherosclerosis. *Cardiovasc Drugs Ther* 2011; **25**: 419–29.

38. Hamilton JA, Myers D, Jessup W, et al. Oxidized LDL can induce macrophage survival, DNA synthesis, and enhanced proliferative response to CSF-1 and GM-CSF. *Arterioscler Thromb Vasc Biol* 1999; **19**: 98–105.

39. Barceló A, Miralles C, Barbe F, et al. Abnormal lipid peroxidation in patients with sleep apnoea. *Eur Respir J* 2000; **16**: 644–7.

40. Kizawa T, Nakamura Y, Takahashi S, et al. Pathogenic role of angiotensin II and oxidised LDL in obstructive sleep apnoea. *Eur Respir J* 2009; **34**: 1390–8.

41. Akinnusi ME, Laporta R, El-Solh AA. Lectin-like oxidized low-density lipoprotein receptor-1 modulates endothelial apoptosis in obstructive sleep apnea. *Chest* 2011; **140**: 1503–10.

42. Tan KC, Chow WS, Lam JC, et al. HDL dysfunction in obstructive sleep apnea. *Atherosclerosis* 2006; **184**: 377–82.

43. Mehra R, Storfer-Isser A, Tracy R, et al. Association of sleep disordered breathing and oxidized LDL. *Am J Respir Crit Care Med* 2010; **181**: A2474.

44. Serebruany V, Sani Y, Eisert C, et al. Effects of Aggrenox and aspirin on plasma endothelial nitric oxide synthase and oxidised low-density lipoproteins in patients after ischaemic stroke. The AGgrenox versus aspirin therapy evaluation (AGATE) biomarker substudy. *Thromb Haemost* 2011; **105**: 81–7.

45. Sarkar PD, Rautaray SS. Oxidized LDL and paraoxanase status in ischemic stroke patients. *Indian J Physiol Pharmacol* 2008; **52**: 403–7.

46. Uno M, Harada M, Takimoto O, et al. Elevation of plasma oxidized LDL in acute stroke patients is associated with ischemic lesions depicted by DWI and predictive of infarct enlargement. *Neurol Res* 2005; **27**: 94–102.

47. Sigurdardottir V, Fagerberg B, Wikstrand J, et al. Circulating oxidized LDL is associated with the occurrence of echolucent plaques in the carotid artery in 61-year-old men. *Scand J Clin Lab Invest* 2008; **68**: 292–7.

48. Shamsuzzaman AS, Winnicki M, Lanfranchi P, et al. Elevated C-reactive protein in patients with obstructive sleep apnea. *Circulation* 2002; **105**: 2462–4.

49. Yokoe T, Minoguchi K, Matsuo H, et al. Elevated levels of C-reactive protein and interleukin-6 in patients with obstructive sleep apnea syndrome are decreased by nasal continuous positive airway pressure. *Circulation* 2003; **107**: 1129–34.

50. Mermigkis C, Bouloukaki I, Mermigkis D, et al. CRP evolution pattern in CPAP-treated obstructive sleep apnea patients.

Does gender play a role? *Sleep Breath* 2012; **16**: 813–19.

51. Sharma SK, Mishra HK, Sharma H, et al. Obesity, and not obstructive sleep apnea, is responsible for increased serum hs-CRP levels in patients with sleep-disordered breathing in Delhi. *Sleep Med* 2008; **9**: 149–56.

52. Firat Guven S, Turkkani MH, Ciftci B, et al. The relationship between high-sensitivity C-reactive protein levels and the severity of obstructive sleep apnea. *Sleep Breath* 2011; **16**: 217–21.

53. Meier-Ewert HK, Ridker PM, Rifai N, et al. Effect of sleep loss on C-reactive protein, an inflammatory marker of cardiovascular risk. *J Am Coll Cardiol* 2004; **43**: 678–83.

54. Lee LA, Chen NH, Huang CG, et al. Patients with severe obstructive sleep apnea syndrome and elevated high-sensitivity C-reactive protein need priority treatment. *Otolaryngol Head Neck Surg* 2010; **143**: 72–7.

55. Lui MM, Lam JC, Mak HK, et al. C-reactive protein is associated with obstructive sleep apnea independent of visceral obesity. *Chest* 2009; **135**: 950–6.

56. Chien MY, Lee P, Tsai YF, et al. C-reactive protein and heart rate recovery in middle-aged men with severe obstructive sleep apnea. *Sleep Breath* 2012; **16**: 629–37.

57. Schiza SE, Mermigkis C, Panagiotis P, et al. C-reactive protein evolution in obstructive sleep apnoea patients under CPAP therapy. *Eur J Clin Invest* 2010; **40**: 968–75.

58. Ford ES, Giles WH. Serum C-reactive protein and self-reported stroke: findings from the Third National Health and Nutrition Examination Survey. *Arterioscler Thromb Vasc Biol* 2000; **20**: 1052–6.

59. Muir KW, Weir CJ, Alwan W, et al. C-reactive protein and outcome after ischemic stroke. *Stroke* 1999; **30**: 981–5.

60. Dziewas R, Ritter M, Kruger L, et al. C-reactive protein and fibrinogen in acute stroke patients with and without sleep apnea. *Cerebrovasc Dis* 2007; **24**: 412–17.

61. Dziewas R, Hopmann B, Humpert M, et al. Capnography screening for sleep apnea in patients with acute stroke. *Neurol Res* 2005; **27**: 83–7.

62. Golbidi S, Badran M, Ayas N, et al. Cardiovascular consequences of sleep apnea. *Lung* 2011; **3**: 3.

63. Jiang Z, Seo JY, Ha H, et al. Reactive oxygen species mediate TGF-beta1-induced plasminogen activator inhibitor-1 upregulation in mesangial cells. *Biochem Biophys Res Commun* 2003; **309**: 961–6.

64. Taddei S, Virdis A, Mattei P, et al. Vascular renin-angiotensin system and sympathetic nervous system activity in human hypertension. *J Cardiovasc Pharmacol* 1994; **23**: S9–14.

65. Shamsuzzaman AS, Somers VK. Fibrinogen, stroke, and obstructive sleep apnea: an evolving paradigm of cardiovascular risk. *Am J Respir Crit Care Med* 2000; **162**: 2018–20.

66. Basoglu OK, Sarac F, Sarac S, et al. Metabolic syndrome, insulin resistance, fibrinogen, homocysteine, leptin, and C-reactive protein in obese patients with obstructive sleep apnea syndrome. *Ann Thorac Med* 2011; **6**: 120–5.

67. Wessendorf TE, Thilmann AF, Wang YM, et al. Fibrinogen levels and obstructive sleep apnea in ischemic stroke. *Am J Respir Crit Care Med* 2000; **162**: 2039–42.

68. Greenberg H, Ye X, Wilson D, et al. Chronic intermittent hypoxia activates nuclear factor-kappaB in cardiovascular tissues in vivo. *Biochem Biophys Res Commun* 2006; **343**: 591–6.

69. Htoo AK, Greenberg H, Tongia S, et al. Activation of nuclear factor kappaB in obstructive sleep apnea: a pathway leading to systemic inflammation. *Sleep Breath* 2006; **10**: 43–50.

70. Dyugovskaya L, Polyakov A, Ginsberg D, et al. Molecular pathways of spontaneous and TNF-{alpha}-mediated neutrophil apoptosis under intermittent hypoxia. *Am J Respir Cell Mol Biol* 2010; **45**: 154–62.

71. Semenza GL. Hypoxia-inducible factor 1 (HIF-1) pathway. *Sci STKE* 2007; **2007**: cm8.

72. Ferrara N, Davis-Smyth T. The biology of vascular endothelial growth factor. *Endocr Rev* 1997; **18**: 4–25.

73. Berger S, Lavie L. Endothelial progenitor cells in cardiovascular disease and hypoxia-potential implications to obstructive sleep apnea. *Transl Res* 2011; **158**: 1–13.

74. Slevin M, Krupinski J, Slowik A, et al. Serial measurement of vascular endothelial growth factor and transforming growth factor-beta1 in serum of patients with acute ischemic stroke. *Stroke* 2000; **31**: 1863–70.

75. Zhang ZG, Chopp M. Neurorestorative therapies for stroke: underlying mechanisms and translation to the clinic. *Lancet Neurol* 2009; **8**: 491–500.

76. Winnicki M, Shamsuzzaman A, Lanfranchi P, et al. Erythropoietin and obstructive sleep apnea. *Am J Hypertens* 2004; **17**: 783–6.

77. Peled N, Kassirer M, Kramer MR, et al. Increased erythrocyte adhesiveness and aggregation in obstructive sleep apnea syndrome. *Thromb Res* 2008; **121**: 631–6.

78. Garvey JF, Taylor CT, McNicholas WT. Cardiovascular disease in obstructive sleep apnoea syndrome: the role of intermittent hypoxia and inflammation. *Eur Respir J* 2009; **33**: 1195–205.

79. Walmsley SR, Print C, Farahi N, et al. Hypoxia-induced neutrophil survival is mediated by HIF-1alpha-dependent NF-kappaB activity. *J Exp Med* 2005; **201**: 105–15.

80. Yuan G, Khan SA, Luo W, et al. Hypoxia-inducible factor 1 mediates increased expression of NADPH oxidase-2 in response to intermittent hypoxia. *J Cell Physiol* 2011; **226**: 2925–33.

81. Lavie L, Polotsky V. Cardiovascular aspects in obstructive sleep apnea syndrome – molecular issues, hypoxia and cytokine profiles. *Respiration* 2009; **78**: 361–70.

82. Alam I, Lewis K, Stephens JW, et al. Obesity, metabolic syndrome and sleep apnoea: all pro-inflammatory states. *Obes Rev* 2007; **8**: 119–27.

83. Minoguchi K, Tazaki T, Yokoe T, et al. Elevated production of tumor necrosis factor-alpha by monocytes in patients with obstructive sleep apnea syndrome. *Chest* 2004; **126**: 1473–9.

84. Dyugovskaya L, Lavie P, Lavie L. Lymphocyte activation as a possible measure of atherosclerotic risk in patients with sleep apnea. *Ann N Y Acad Sci* 2005; **1051**: 340–50.

85. Arias MA, García-Río F, Alonso-Fernández A, et al. CPAP decreases plasma levels of soluble tumour necrosis factor-alpha receptor 1 in obstructive sleep apnoea. *Eur Respir J* 2008; **32**: 1009–15.

86. Rodondi N, Marques-Vidal P, Butler J, et al. Markers of atherosclerosis and inflammation for prediction of coronary heart disease in older adults. *Am J Epidemiol* 2010; **171**: 540–9.

87. Zaremba J, Losy J. Early TNF-alpha levels correlate with ischaemic stroke severity. *Acta Neurol Scand* 2001; **104**: 288–95.

88. Vila N, Castillo J, Dávalos A, et al. Levels of anti-inflammatory cytokines and neurological worsening in acute ischemic stroke. *Stroke* 2003; **34**: 671–5.

89. Varadhachary AS, Monestier M, Salgame P. Reciprocal induction of IL-10 and IL-12 from macrophages by low-density lipoprotein and its oxidized forms. *Cell Immunol* 2001; **213**: 45–51.

90. Koutsourelakis I, Vagiakis E, Perraki E, et al. Nasal inflammation in sleep apnoea patients using CPAP and effect of heated humidification. *Eur Respir J* 2011; **37**: 587–94.

91. Zaremba J, Losy J. Interleukin-12 in acute ischemic stroke patients. *Folia Neuropathol* 2006; **44**: 59–66.

92. Ormstad H, Aass HC, Lund-Sorensen N, et al. Serum levels of cytokines and C-reactive protein in acute ischemic stroke patients, and their relationship to stroke lateralization, type, and infarct volume. *J Neurol* 2011; **258**: 677–85.

93. Tailor A, Granger DN. Role of adhesion molecules in vascular regulation and damage. *Curr Hypertens Rep* 2000; **2**: 78–83.

94. Quehenberger O. Thematic review series: the immune system and atherogenesis. Molecular mechanisms regulating monocyte recruitment in atherosclerosis. *J Lipid Res* 2005; **46**: 1582–90.

95. Lavie L. Oxidative stress–a unifying paradigm in obstructive sleep apnea and comorbidities. *Prog Cardiovasc Dis* 2009; **51**: 303–12.

96. Budhiraja R, Budhiraja P, Quan SF. Sleep-disordered breathing and cardiovascular disorders. *Respir Care* 2010; **55**: 1322–32.

97. El-Solh AA, Mador MJ, Sikka P, et al. Adhesion molecules in patients with coronary artery disease and moderate-to-severe obstructive sleep apnea. *Chest* 2002; **121**: 1541–7.

98. Cofta S, Wysocka E, Michalak S, et al. Endothelium-derived markers and antioxidant status in the blood of obstructive sleep apnea males. *Eur J Med Res* 2009; **14**: 49–52.

99. Shimizu M, Kamio K, Haida M, et al. Platelet activation in patients with obstructive sleep apnea syndrome and effects of nasal-continuous positive airway pressure. *Tokai J Exp Clin Med* 2002; **27**: 107–12.

100. Ishikawa M, Cooper D, Arumugam TV, et al. Platelet-leukocyte-endothelial cell interactions after middle cerebral artery occlusion and reperfusion. *J Cereb Blood Flow Metab* 2004; **24**: 907–15.

101. Ajjan R, Kearney MT, Grant PJ. Insulin resistance and the pathogenesis of cardiovascular disease. In: Zeitler PS, Nadeau KJ, eds. *Insulin Resistance: Childhood Precursors and Adult Disease.* Totowa, NJ: Humana Press, 2008, 179–205.

102. Budhiraja R, Parthasarathy S, Quan SF. Endothelial dysfunction in obstructive sleep apnea. *J Clin Sleep Med* 2007; **3**: 409–15.

103. Anderson TJ. Nitric oxide, atherosclerosis and the clinical relevance of endothelial dysfunction. *Heart Fail Rev* 2003; **8**: 71–86.

104. Lavie L. Sleep apnea syndrome, endothelial dysfunction, and cardiovascular morbidity. *Sleep* 2004; **27**: 1053–5.

105. Itzhaki S, Lavie L, Pillar G, et al. Endothelial dysfunction in obstructive sleep apnea measured by peripheral arterial tone response in the finger to reactive hyperemia. *Sleep* 2005; **28**: 594–600.

106. Itzhaki S, Dorchin H, Clark G, et al. The effects of 1-year treatment with a herbst mandibular advancement splint on obstructive sleep apnea, oxidative stress, and endothelial function. *Chest* 2007; **131**: 740–9.

107. Jelic S, Lederer DJ, Adams T, et al. Endothelial repair capacity and apoptosis are inversely related in obstructive sleep apnea. *Vasc Health Risk Manag* 2009; **5**: 909–20.

108. Freestone B, Chong AY, Nuttall S, et al. Impaired flow mediated dilatation as evidence of endothelial dysfunction in chronic atrial fibrillation: relationship to plasma von Willebrand factor and soluble E-selectin levels. *Thromb Res* 2008; **122**: 85–90.

109. Kheirandish-Gozal L, Bhattacharjee R, Kim J, et al. Endothelial progenitor cells and vascular dysfunction in children with obstructive sleep apnea. *Am J Respir Crit Care Med* 2010; **182**: 92–7.

110. Butt M, Khair OA, Dwivedi G, et al. Myocardial perfusion by myocardial contrast echocardiography and endothelial dysfunction in obstructive sleep apnea. *Hypertension* 2011; **58**: 417–24.

111. Sobrino T, Hurtado O, Moro MA, et al. The increase of circulating endothelial progenitor cells after acute ischemic stroke is associated with good outcome. *Stroke* 2007; **38**: 2759–64.

112. Fan Y, Shen F, Frenzel T, et al. Endothelial progenitor cell transplantation improves long-term stroke outcome in mice. *Ann Neurol* 2010; **67**: 488–97.

113. Levy P, Pepin JL, Arnaud C, et al. Obstructive sleep apnea and atherosclerosis. *Prog Cardiovasc Dis* 2009; **51**: 400–10.

114. Suzuki T, Nakano H, Maekawa J, et al. Obstructive sleep apnea and carotid-artery intima-media thickness. *Sleep* 2004; **27**: 129–33.

115. Baguet JP, Hammer L, Levy P, et al. The severity of oxygen desaturation is predictive of carotid wall thickening and plaque occurrence. *Chest* 2005; **128**: 3407–12.

116. Turmel J, Series F, Boulet LP, et al. Relationship between atherosclerosis and the sleep apnea syndrome: an intravascular ultrasound study. *Int J Cardiol* 2009; **132**: 203–9.

117. Drager LF, Bortolotto LA, Figueiredo AC, et al. Effects of continuous positive airway pressure on early signs of atherosclerosis in obstructive sleep apnea. *Am J Respir Crit Care Med* 2007; **176**: 706–12.

118. Drager LF, Polotsky VY, Lorenzi-Filho G. Obstructive sleep apnea: an emerging risk factor for atherosclerosis. *Chest* 2011; **140**: 534–42.

119. Dziewas R, Ritter M, Usta N, et al. Atherosclerosis and obstructive sleep apnea in patients with ischemic stroke. *Cerebrovasc Dis* 2007; **24**: 122–6.

120. Steiner S, Schueller PO, Schulze V, et al. Occurrence of coronary collateral vessels in patients with sleep apnea and total coronary occlusion. *Chest* 2010; **137**: 516–20.

121. Lavie P, Lavie L, Herer P. All-cause mortality in males with sleep apnoea syndrome: declining mortality rates with age. *Eur Respir J* 2005; **25**: 514–20.

122. Lavie P, Lavie L. Unexpected survival advantage in elderly people with moderate sleep apnoea. *J Sleep Res* 2009; **18**: 397–403.

123. Lavie L, Lavie P. Ischemic preconditioning as a possible explanation for the age decline relative mortality in sleep apnea. *Med Hypotheses* 2006; **66**: 1069–73.

Chapter 3

Sleep apnea, autonomic dysfunction, and vascular diseases

Pietro Cortelli and Federica Provini

Synopsis

Habitual snoring and obstructive sleep apnea syndrome (OSAS) are common respiratory disorders affecting up to 10% of the population.

Obstructive sleep apnea syndrome is characterized by recurrent episodes of complete or partial interruption of ventilation during sleep, caused by collapse of the upper airways.

Compared with the general population, the prevalence of OSAS is higher among patients with cardio- and cerebrovascular conditions. About 50% of OSA patients are hypertensive and about 30% of hypertensive patients also have obstructive sleep apneas (OSAs).

Epidemiological data indicate that OSA is involved in the development or progression of cardio- and cerebrovascular diseases.

Obstructive sleep apnea has been recognized as a risk factor for the onset of arterial hypertension, coronary artery disease, heart failure, and stroke, independent of confounding covariates (i.e., age, gender, smoking, alcohol, obesity, diabetes, or dyslipidemia).

The underlying mechanisms explaining the association between OSA and cardio- and cerebrovascular diseases have not been fully defined.

Sympathetic overactivity appears to be the critical link between OSA and the pathogenesis of hypertension, as documented by clinical studies and strong experimental evidence from animal studies.

Several intermediate mechanisms, including oxidative stress, disorders in coagulation factors, endothelial dysfunction, platelet activation, and increased inflammatory processes have also been implicated in the pathogenesis of cardio- and cerebrovascular diseases.

The purpose of this chapter is to discuss the interactions between OSAS and cardio- and cerebrovascular diseases, focusing on the mechanisms by which OSA may contribute to the onset and progression of cardiovascular diseases.

Introduction

Obstructive sleep apnea syndrome is the most common form of sleep-disordered breathing, affecting approximately 4% of men and 2% of women in the general population [1]. Obstructive sleep apnea syndrome can occur at all ages, but the incidence is highest among the middle-aged.

Obstructive sleep apnea syndrome is characterized by habitual and intensely loud snoring intermingled with repetitive partial (hypopnea) or complete (apnea) upper airway obstruction during sleep, associated with increasing respiratory efforts, intermittent arterial oxygen

Sleep, Stroke, and Cardiovascular Disease, ed. Antonio Culebras. Published by Cambridge University Press. © Cambridge University Press 2013.

desaturation, systemic and pulmonary arterial blood pressure surges, and sleep disruption. These cycles may occur hundreds of times a night in a patient with moderate to severe OSAS, and the frequency of apneas and hypopneas is usually expressed as the number of upper airway obstructions per hour of sleep (the apnea/hypopnea index).

In addition to causing nonrestorative sleep and excessive daytime sleepiness, considerable evidence is available of an independent association between OSAS, systemic hypertension, and cardio- and cerebrovascular diseases [2–10].

The mechanisms underlying the development of cardiovascular disease in OSA patients are not completely understood but they are likely to be multifactorial, including the direct effects of intermittent hypoxemia and hypercapnia on chemoreceptors and sympathethic nervous system (SNS) activity [11,12], changes to the cardiovascular system (including fluid balance) in response to marked fluctuations in intrathoracic pressure during obstructive apneas, the generalized stress from sleep disruption (the arousal effect), and other less-known factors such as selective activation of inflammatory pathways, endothelial dysfunction, abnormal coagulation, and metabolic and endocrinological dysregulation.

Whatever the mechanism underlying the dangerous association between OSA and cardiovascular disease, it is very important to recognize patients with cardiovascular disease who have coexisting sleep apnea and to understand the possible reversible mechanisms by which sleep apnea may contribute to the progression of the cardiovascular condition to implement effective treatment strategies.

This chapter focuses on the interactions between OSAS and cardio- and cerebrovascular diseases, and particularly on the autonomic mechanisms by which OSA may contribute to the onset and progression of cardiovascular diseases.

Sleep and autonomic nervous system interactions

Through its complex central and peripheral circuits, the autonomic nervous system (ANS) controls vital involuntary functions of the body such as circulation, respiration, thermoregulation, neuroendocrine secretion, and gastrointestinal and genitourinary functions. The ANS is closely related to sleep from anatomical, physiological and neurochemical points of view, resulting in dynamic synchronous fluctuations in sleep phases and autonomic functions. Sleep state changes are coordinated principally by the pons, basal forebrain areas, and other subcortical structures, and the main neurotransmitters are norephinephrine, serotonin, and acetylcholine. Through its ascending and descending connections between the hypothalamic–limbic region and the nucleus tractus solitarius in the medulla, the central autonomic network orchestrates the two efferent divisions of the ANS (sympathetic and parasympathetic). Sleep induces profound changes in ANS functions and ANS disorders affect vital functioning during sleep, including circulation and respiration. Non-rapid eye movement (NREM) sleep is characterized by electrocortical synchronization, reduced muscle tone, and stable parasympathetic predominance. Breathing and cardiocirculatory monitoring document a progressive deactivation from stage 1 to stage 3 NREM sleep. During light sleep, these functions alternate phases of activation and deactivation every 20 to 40 seconds [13].

All these changes suggest an increased sensitivity of the baroreceptor reflex that contributes to the reduced variability of arterial pressure typical of NREM sleep [14,15]. In NREM sleep, sympathetic activity may be transiently increased by arousal stimuli, coinciding with the appearance of K complexes in the electroencephalogram. This is associated with increased heart rate and respiration. During NREM sleep respiration is controlled by an automatic system localized in the medulla that is activated by chemical stimuli.

Rapid eye movement (REM) sleep is characterized by electrocortical desynchronization, muscle atonia, and phasic motor autonomic changes. Autonomic function during REM sleep is characterized by marked phasic fluctuations of sympathetic and parasympathetic activity and impairment of baroreflex responses and thermoregulation. During tonic REM sleep there is a marked bradycardia and decreased peripheral resistance, resulting in a decrease in arterial pressure interrupted by large transient increases in arterial pressure and heart rate during bursts of rapid eye movements and muscle twitches. This is the result of phasic inhibition of parasympathetic activity and phasic increases in sympathetic discharge. Irregularity in breathing is typical of REM sleep and is caused by the extremely variable behavior of medullary respiratory neurons during this stage. Some studies have shown that the central respiratory drive, although erratic, is often increased in REM sleep. It is also known that medullary respiratory activity in REM sleep is influenced by at least one type of phasic REM sleep event, the pontine–geniculate–occipital spikes wave, a finding clearly indicating nonrespiratory and state-specific influences on the respiratory system in REM sleep. Nocturnal monitoring of breathing, pulse rate, systemic arterial pressure, and peripheral vasomotor activation discloses autonomic deactivation that, appearing at sleep onset, continues into deep sleep. Marked autonomic reactivation characterizes REM sleep. These autonomic patterns broadly fit the idea that NREM sleep corresponds to a deactivation of brain functions, whereas REM sleep is the outcome of an endogenous brain reactivation.

However, not all autonomic activities have the same nocturnal trend. Spontaneous sympathetic skin responses (SSRs) are particularly abundant during deep (stage 3) sleep when breathing and cardiocirculatory systems stabilize at a minimum level of activities and evoked SSRs are markedly inhibited in NREM and REM sleep, even though breathing and circulation behave differently in these two types of sleep [16].

The study of regional blood flow (and, hence, metabolism and synaptic activities) confirms that the functional state of the brain during sleep is not merely oriented toward activation (REM sleep) or deactivation (NREM sleep). In deep sleep, for example, there are cortical areas (e.g., the hippocampus) and subcortical areas (e.g., the amygdala) that are directly involved in the autonomic expression of emotion, and maintain a flow (and, hence, a functional level) similar to that of wakefulness [17].

The characteristics of thermoregulatory control vary significantly between sleep phases and wakefulness and with time of the day, being modulated by the circadian system and sleep control mechanisms. Body temperature is regulated at a lower level during NREM sleep than during wakefulness, with a decrease in body temperature and metabolism. Thermoregulatory responses to changes in peripheral or core temperature in animal studies show qualitatively different responses in NREM compared to REM sleep. During NREM sleep thermoregulation mechanisms are operative and the ambient thermal load variations are balanced. This homeothermy is controlled by hypothalamic–preoptic integrative mechanisms that drive subordinate brainstem and spinal somatic and visceral mechanisms. By contrast, the transition from NREM sleep to REM sleep is characterized by disruption of ongoing thermoregulation that is mostly suspended in REM sleep. In this phase there is a marked inhibition of thermoregulation and the changes in body temperature occur passively in relation to the heat environmental load. The result is that body temperature changes according to its thermal inertia [18]. On the other hand, thermal environment and body temperature are important determinants of sleep architecture having a prominent influence on both the amount and distribution of arousal states. In particular, some studies have shown that in a cold environment there is an increase in wakefulness, sleep latency, and movement time, and the decrease in sleep time is mostly due to decreased REM sleep and stage 2 of NREM sleep [19].

Hormones have a mutually regulatory influence on circadian rhythms and the sleep–wake cycle. Melatonin levels are higher during night sleep; cortisol is low at the usual sleep onset, but then it is high at the habitual morning wake-up time. The thyroid stimulating hormone peak in the middle of the night is blunted by sleep; growth hormone, prolactin, and parathyroid hormone show a prominent sleep-related increase in levels. Renin levels are augmented in stage 3 of NREM sleep.

The hemodynamic consequences of sleep apnea

In their pioneering studies published in the *Bulletin de Physiopathologie Respiratoire*, Coccagna et al. and Lugaresi et al. first used invasive blood pressure monitoring to document the dramatic hemodynamic consequences of sleep apnea in sleeping OSAS patients [20,21]. They described the transient cardiovascular changes that accompany OSA events: heart rate (HR), systemic blood pressure (BP), and pulmonary arterial pressure initially decline with the onset of apnea and rise acutely with its termination.

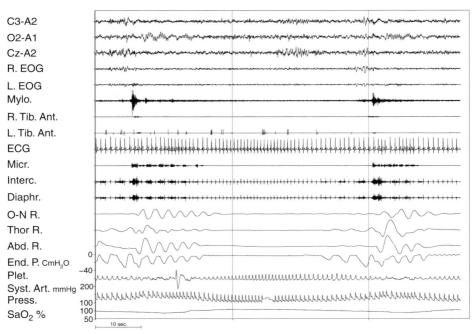

Figure 3.1. Mixed (central and obstructive) sleep apnea. Initially the apnea is central with a cessation of nasal, thoracic, and abdominal respiration. In the second part of the apnea, during upper airway obstruction intercostal and diaphragmatic muscle activity increases progressively, being associated with wide variations in endoesophageal negative pressure, indicating great expiratory effort. Heart rate and systemic arterial pressure initially fall and subsequently rise acutely with apnea termination. C3-A2, O2-A1, Cz-A2, electroencephalogram; R, right; L, left; EOG, electrooculogram; Mylo., mylohyoideus muscle; Tib. Ant., tibialis anterior muscle; ECG, electrocardiogram; Micr., microphone; Interc., intercostalis muscle; Diaphr., diaphragm muscle; O-N R., oral-nasal respiration; Thor., thoracic; Abd., abdominal; End. P., intraesophageal pressure; Plet., plethysmogram; System. Art. Press., systemic arterial pressure; SaO2, oxyhemoglobin saturation.

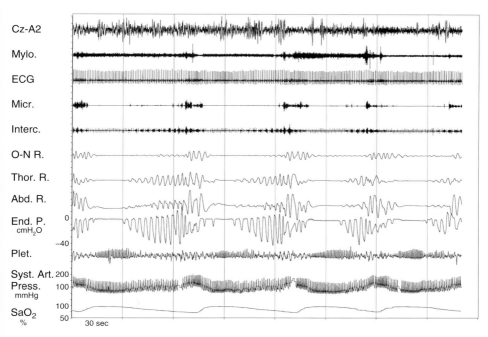

Figure 3.2. Repetitive cardiorespiratory modifications induced by an interrupted series of obstructive sleep apneas, which causes a complex autonomic response characterized by initial parasympathetic predominance followed by a surge of sympathetic activity with arousal and a sudden increase in BP and HR. Cz-A2, electroencephalogram; Mylo., mylohyoideus muscle; ECG, electrocardiogram; Micr., microphone; Interc., intercostalis muscle; O-N R., oral-nasal respiration; Thor., thoracic; Abd., abdominal; End. P., intraesophageal pressure; Plet., plethysmogram; System. Art. Press., systemic arterial pressure; SaO$_2$, oxyhemoglobin saturation.

Surges in HR and BP typically occur 5 to 7 seconds after apnea termination, coinciding with arousal from sleep, peak ventilation, and the nadir of oxyhemoglobin saturation (SaO$_2$) (Figure 3.1). In patients with severe OSAS, BP may reach 200/100 mmHg, lasting a few seconds in the recovery phase from apnea; arterial SaO$_2$ often falls below 70% (Figure 3.2). As a consequence of the repetitive obstructive apneas, hemodynamic variables and cardiovascular autonomic activity oscillate continuously between the apneic and ventilatory phases, resulting in increasing BP variability and average BP level [22] (Figure 3.3). These continuous surges in HR and BP during the night counteract the usual fall in HR and BP that accompany normal sleep and the absence of the normal decrease in blood pressure during sleep termed nondipping [22]. In a representative population of male essential hypertensive nondippers, we used polysomnography to document the absence of sleep-related BP decline and increased BP variability in 10 out of 11 apneic snorers [23,24]. Hence underdiagnosed apneic snoring could play an important role in determining changes in the circadian BP profile toward nondipping, while repeated bouts of hypertension night after night in patients with untreated sleep apnea may eventually lead to sustained 24-hour hypertension. In fact, half or more of all OSAS patients are hypertensive, not only during nighttime sleep but also during daytime activity, and several studies have found an approximately 30% prevalence of OSAS among patients with "primary" hypertension [25].

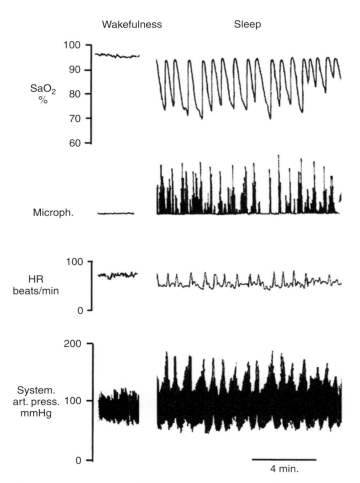

Figure 3.3. Continuous marked increases in systemic arterial pressure (System. art. press.) and heart rate (HR) during an interrupted series of obstructive sleep apneas (see oxyhemoglobin saturation (SaO₂) falls, associated with the cessation of snoring on the microphone (Microph.) trace).

Heart rate variability

Obstructive sleep apnea influences heart rate variability, a well-established marker of cardiovascular risk not only during sleep but also during wakefulness. Analysis of the circadian rhythm of heart rate variability shows that the mean high-frequency value (parasympathetic activity index) from morning to noon is lower, whereas the mean low-frequency/high-frequency ratio (sympathetic activity index) is higher in OSAS patients than in controls [26].

In 1994, Cortelli and coworkers demonstrated that normotensive OSAS patients have higher heart rate and norepinephrine plasma levels at rest during wakefulness and a higher blood pressure response to head-up tilt compared to controls, suggesting sympathetic overactivity [27]. Further, when performing cardiovascular reflex tests, OSAS patients showed significantly lower values of respiratory arrhythmia and Valsalva ratio (Figure 3.4) associated with a greater decrease in heart rate induced by the cold face test, indicating a blunting of

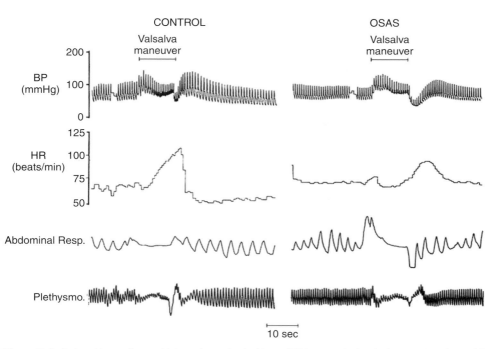

Figure 3.4. Reduced baroreflex sensitivity as shown by the blunted HR increase during the hypotensive phase of the Valsalva maneuver in patients with OSAS compared to controls. OSAS, obstructive sleep apnea syndrome; BP, blood pressure; HR, heart rate; Resp., respirogram; Plethysmo., plethysmogram.

reflexes dependent on baroreceptor or pulmonary afferents and normal or increased cardiac vagal efferent activity (Figure 3.5).

An imbalance in the autonomic regulation of heart rate after maximal exercise, characterized by an attenuated heart rate recovery, has also been documented in OSA patients compared to overweight and normal weight controls [28].

In addition, studies of heart rate variability using spectral analysis show sympathetic activation (increased low-frequency component and increased low-frequency/high-frequency ratio) during sleep apnea episodes [29–31].

Treatment of OSA with continuous positive airway pressure (CPAP) leads to a significant improvement of autonomic modulation and cardiovascular variability [32].

The autonomic consequences of sleep apnea: sympathetic activation

With its continuous repetition of obstructive events during the night, OSAS is a paradigm of how a sleep breathing disorder can translate into a permanent dysregulation of the autonomic control of the cardiovascular system, resulting in sympathetic overactivity. Whatever the causal factors, the increase in sympathetic tone in relation to the apneic episodes is believed to be the possible determinant of cardiovascular complications that also account for the increased risk of mortality in patients with sleep apnea [27,33,34]. Microneurography, a technique evaluating autonomic discharges in nerves, has shown increased muscle sympathetic nervous activity

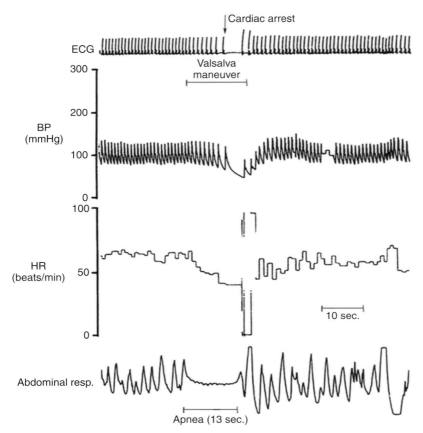

Figure 3.5. The exaggerated HR response to the association of a voluntary apnea and the cold face test leading, in some cases, to a cardiac arrest in obstructive sleep apnea patients. This peculiar combination of reduced baroreflex and hyperactive chemoreflex suggests that a central remodeling of the autonomic control of the cardiovascular system may precede the development of diurnal hypertension. ECG, electrocardiogram; BP, blood pressure; HR, heart rate; Resp., respiration.

(MSNA) in patients with OSA compared to controls [35]. Obstructive sleep apnea syndrome patients with hypertension responded favorably to CPAP treatment, that also led to a marked fall in daytime MSNA [36].

Among the pathogenetic mechanisms underlying the increased sympathetic activity, intermittent hypoxia and changes in ventilation mechanics together with arousals due to the activation of cortical and subcortical structures have been implicated as important determinants, although this topic remains a matter of debate. The pathogenetic link between OSAS and increased sympathetic activity appears to be more complex and multifactorial in nature, as all previous studies showed the contribution of several mechanisms in the complex relation between these putative autonomic factors and the cardiovascular complications of OSAS.

Intermittent hypoxia can drive the sympathoexcitation that accompanies OSAS but its role is controversial. Reduced blood oxygen tension stimulates the peripheral arterial chemoreceptors, increasing sympathetic activity with consequent acute increases in arterial blood pressure [37].

However, some authors emphasize that the chemoreflex response to hypoxia cannot be entirely responsible for the acute autonomic effects of sleep apnea, because elimination of hypoxia only modestly dampens the HR and BP oscillations that accompany OSA [38]. The same authors suggested that hypercapnia is a more potent stimulus for sympathoexcitation than hypoxia itself, causing increased ventilation, tachycardia, cardiac output, and BP.

Support for the role of sympathetic overactivity in the pathogenesis of hypertension in OSAS also comes from animal models of OSA, in which an intact sympathetic system was required for the animals to manifest increased blood pressure. An increase in blood pressure was found in both dog and rat models of OSAS; blood pressure declined once the airway occlusion or intermittent hypoxia was abolished [12,39]. These blood pressure changes were not observed with induced recurrent arousals without airway occlusion, indicating that the obstructive events rather than the associated arousals were responsible for the observed effects [39].

Obstructive sleep apnea and baroreflex function

Narkiewicz and colleagues showed that normotensive patients with OSA have a selective impairment of the sympathetic response to baroreceptor stimulation, apparently not accompanied by any impairment of baroreflex control of HR [40]. Conversely, by assessing "spontaneous" baroreflex sensitivity through the sequence method, Parati et al., Bonsignore et al., and Lombardi et al. reported a clearcut impairment of baroreflex control of HR, mostly evident during NREM sleep in OSAS patients [41–44].

The first study aiming to identify markers for the development of future daytime hypertension in a group of OSAS patients, still normotensive during the day at baseline, showed that a reduced baroreflex sensitivity plus a hyperactive chemoreflex were characteristic features of OSAS in the awake state. This peculiar combination of reduced baroreflex and hyperactive chemoreflex function suggested that a central remodeling of the autonomic control of the cardiovascular system may precede the development of daytime hypertension [27].

Chronic intermittent hypoxia, associated with recurrent apneas, exerts two major effects on the carotid body, including sensitization of the hypoxic sensory response and induction of sensory long-term facilitation. Studies in humans and experimental models suggest that alterations in acute O_2 sensing by the carotid bodies and hyperactivity of adrenal medullary chromaffin cells both contribute to the autonomic comorbidities associated with chronic intermittent hypoxia [38], inducing activation of specific transcription factors and alterations in gene expression associated with increased oxidative stress [45].

Moreover, preliminary results reported by Cortelli et al. [27] were confirmed in the awake state by Carlson in 1996 and Narkiewicz in 1998, using different methods of baroreflex sensitivity index (BRSI) computation, also showing that the reduced BRSI of OSAS patients is independent of hypertension, obesity, and age [40,46]. These conclusions are in line with the autonomic data obtained during sleep by Bonsignore et al. and Parati et al. These studies evaluated BRSI with the sequence technique and found the index was also depressed during sleep, particularly during stage 2 of NREM, and this alteration was reversed with the treatment of OSA with CPAP [41,47].

Thus a reduced BRSI is a feature of OSAS before the appearance of cardiovascular complications. Whether other mechanisms (e.g., chemoreflex activation, sleep fragmentation, humoral changes, etc.) also contribute to a sustained daytime hypertensive condition, starting from repeated episodic apnea-related surges of nocturnal blood pressure, is still a matter of investigation.

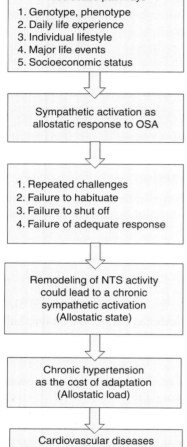

OSA

Prediseae pathways
1. Genotype, phenotype
2. Daily life experience
3. Individual lifestyle
4. Major life events
5. Socioeconomic status

Sympathetic activation as allostatic response to OSA

1. Repeated challenges
2. Failure to habituate
3. Failure to shut off
4. Failure of adequate response

Remodeling of NTS activity could lead to a chronic sympathetic activation (Allostatic state)

Chronic hypertension as the cost of adaptation (Allostatic load)

Cardiovascular diseases

Figure 3.6. The diagram depicts the allostatic interpretation of the transformation of episodic hypertensive peaks associated with obstructive sleep apnea (OSA) into a sustained 24-hour hypertension. In predisposed obstructive sleep apnea syndrome subjects, repeated long periods of allostatic sympathetic activation required to interrupt the dangerous apnea may cause a remodeling of nucleus tractus solitarii (NTS) activity. This occurs by means of nocturnal stimulation of the baro- and chemoreflex visceral afferents, leading to a cascade effect on the ventrolateral medulla that may be responsible for the sustained chronic peripheral sympathetic overactivation.

This host of phenomena could be better understood from an allostatic perspective. In this view, the allostatic sympathetic activation functional to the characteristic respiratory and cardiovascular effects of OSAs, when repeated over a long period in predisposed subjects, may induce a further remodeling of nucleus tractus solitarii (NTS) activity (Figure 3.6). Repeated nocturnal episodic stimulation of the baro- and chemoreflex visceral afferents could lead to a cascade effect on the ventrolateral medulla, which could in turn be responsible for the sustained chronic peripheral sympathetic overactivation. Thus, the chronic hypertensive state associated with OSAS might be viewed from the allostatic perspective as the cost of ANS adaptation to the episodic recurrence of sympathetic surges during the night. From this standpoint, the reduced BRSI described consistently in OSAS could therefore be an indirect index of this maladaptive process.

On the basis of this hypothesis and considering that none of the markers of oxygen desaturation and sleep disruption were also correlated with excessive daytime somnolence

(EDS), a disabling chronic complication of OSAS, a study was undertaken to explore the occurrence of EDS in untreated subjects with sleep-related breathing disorders (SRBDs) of different severity in relation to cardiac autonomic modulation [43].

Excessive daytime somnolence was diagnosed objectively by the multiple sleep latency test (MSLT) in a cohort of 53 subjects with SRBD who underwent nocturnal polysomnography (PSG). The BRSI was measured by the sequence technique and the cardiac sympathovagal balance by power spectral analysis of whole-night ECG and continuous BP recordings separately over each sleep phase. The PSG indices of the severity of SRBD and quality of sleep were computed and correlated with the autonomic cardiac indices.

Patients without EDS (nEDS group) and patients with EDS (EDS group) were matched for age, BMI, resting BP value, and habitual consumption of alcohol, caffeine, and nicotine. No significant differences were found in sleep quality or sleep structure between the nEDS and EDS groups. In addition, nighttime values of BP and HR and lowest oxygen saturation were similar in the EDS and nEDS groups.

Hence, this study failed to explain EDS by any of these variables. However, analyzing the baroreflex sensitivity (BRS) and the cardiac sympatho/vagal balance, patients with EDS had a reduced BRS and an increased low frequency/high frequency (LF/HF) ratio, which is believed to be a marker of sympathetic activity. Moreover, the impaired modulation of BRS and the LF/HF ratio among the various sleep stages was significantly more evident in patients with EDS, suggesting that patients with SRBD and EDS have a reduced BRS and an increased sympatho/vagal balance over the whole night, with an impaired modulation of the LF/HF power ratio among the sleep stages [43].

Although this study did not demonstrate a causal link between reduced BRS, altered cardiac autonomic modulation, and EDS due to its cross-sectional nature, the autonomic impairment found in EDS patients may suggest a possible contribution by EDS to the increased rate of cardiovascular events in patients with SRBD. It may also indicate that exploring cardiac autonomic modulation during the night might help to identify patients with SRBD at risk for EDS. In turn, given the known prognostic value of alterations in cardiac autonomic modulation, assessment of autonomic function in these patients may help to identify one of the mechanisms potentially associated with an increased cardiovascular risk in this condition.

This hypothesis was recently supported by a cross-sectional multicenter study on 6046 subjects from the Sleep Heart Health Study. The results demonstrated that the association of sleep-disordered breathing (SDB) with hypertension is stronger in individuals who report daytime sleepiness than in those who do not, unequivocally indicating the importance of taking the level of daytime somnolence into account to prevent cardiovascular events in patients with SRBD [48].

This hypothesis may be indirectly supported by short-term studies failing to show any hypotensive effect of CPAP on 24-hour ambulatory blood pressure in patients with severe OSAS but without EDS [49,50]. However, a small decrease in blood pressure values in non-sleepy patients with OSAS may be observed over longer follow-up periods. Indeed, Barbé et al. showed a BP reduction in treated OSA patients only after one year of CPAP treatment and only in patients who used the CPAP for more than five to six hours per night [51,52].

A recent study described the characteristics of residual excessive sleepiness (RES) in OSA patients adequately treated with CPAP [53], but failed to prove an association with altered cardiac autonomic modulation, suggesting that RES may have multifactorial causes [54].

Other less well-assessed risk factors in obstructive sleep apnea

More recently, other less well-assessed risk factors have been implicated in the pathogenesis of cardiovascular complications in sleep apnea.

The vascular system/endothelium, recognized to be a biologically active system maintaining the balance between vasodilation and vasoconstriction, may be dysfunctional in OSA and may be an important marker of cardiovascular risk [55]. Endothelial dysfunction has been found to occur in response to cardiovascular risk factors and to precede or accelerate the development of atherosclerosis. The endothelium also produces vasoconstrictor substances, such as endothelin and angiotensin II, and their levels have been reported to increase in OSAS, although not invariably.

Recent observations have led to a hypothesis that OSA may trigger an inflammatory–metabolic syndrome. Obstructive sleep apnea-induced hypoxic stress can modulate circulating proinflammatory mediators, causing accelerated atherogenesis, prothrombotic coagulation shifts, and increased platelet aggregation. In fact, various endocrine and cytokine alterations are observed in SDB patients, such as increases in interleukin-6, tumor necrosis factor, C-reactive protein, adhesion molecules, leptin, and insulin, independent of obesity or age [56].

Another link between the mechanism of hypertension and OSA is the renin–angiotensin system. Patients with OSA demonstrate increased renin–angiotensin activity that improves with treatment [57].

However, such a conclusion needs to be made with caution because of the confounding effects of comorbidities. Indeed, endothelial dysfunction is often seen in patients with hypertension, hyperlipidemia, diabetes, or smoking, and these associations may limit the importance of OSAS as an independent risk factor for endothelial or inflammatory dysfunction, an issue that deserves further investigation by studies including larger numbers of patients, and adequately controlled for potential confounding factors [44].

Conclusions

All the evidence gathered to date supports the importance of viewing the effect of OSA on the cardiovascular system from an autonomic standpoint. Measuring ANS function by means of "spontaneous" baroreflex cardiac modulation or other methods may not only help recognize the severity and prognostic relevance of the cardiovascular effect of OSA, but also shed light on the pathophysiological mechanisms that transform transient nocturnal alterations into sustained 24-hour derangements that require treatment.

References

1. Young T, Palta M, Dempsey J, et al. The occurrence of sleep-disordered breathing among middle-aged adults. *N Engl J Med* 1993; **328**: 1230–5.

2. Lugaresi E, Cirignotta F, Coccagna G, et al. Some epidemiological data on snoring and cardiocirculatory disturbances. *Sleep* 1980; **3**: 221–4.

3. Partinen M, Guilleminault C. Daytime sleepiness and vascular morbidity at seven-year follow-up in obstructive sleep apnea patients. *Chest* 1990; **97**: 27–32.

4. Young T, Shahar E, Nieto FJ, et al. Predictors of sleep-disordered breathing in community-dwelling adults: the Sleep Heart Health Study. *Arch Intern Med* 2002; **162**: 893–900.

5. Nieto FJ, Young TB, Lind BK, et al. Association of sleep disordered breathing, sleep apnea, and hypertension in a large

community-based study. Sleep Heart Health Study. *JAMA* 2000; **283**: 1829–36.

6. Peppard PE, Young T, Palta M, et al. Prospective study of the association between sleep-disordered breathing and hypertension. *N Engl J Med* 2000; **342**: 1378–84.

7. Lavie P, Herer P, Hoffstein V. Obstructive sleep apnoea syndrome as a risk factor for hypertension: population study. *BMJ* 2000; **320**: 479–82.

8. Somers VK, White DP, Amin R, et al. Sleep apnea and cardiovascular disease: an American Heart Association/American College of Cardiology Foundation Scientific Statement from the American Heart Association Council for High Blood Pressure Research Professional Education Committee, Council on Clinical Cardiology, Stroke Council, and Council on Cardiovascular Nursing. *J Am Coll Cardiol* 2008; **52**: 686–717.

9. Bassetti C, Aldrich MS. Sleep apnea in acute cerebrovascular diseases: final report on 128 patients. *Sleep* 1999; **22**: 217–23.

10. Yaggi HK, Concato J, Kernan WN, et al. Obstructive sleep apnea as a risk factor for stroke and death. *N Engl J Med* 2005; **353**: 2034–41.

11. Fletcher EC. An animal model of the relationship between systemic hypertension and repetitive episodic hypoxia as seen in sleep apnoea. *J Sleep Res* 1995; **4**: 71–7.

12. Flectcher EC. Physiological consequences of intermittent hypoxia: systemic blood pressure. *J Appl Physiol* 2001; **90**: 1600–5.

13. Lugaresi E, Coccagna G, Mantovani M, et al. Some periodic phenomena arising during drowsiness and sleep in man. *Electroencephalogr Clin Neurophysiol* 1972; **32**: 701–5.

14. Conway J, Boon N, Jones JV, et al. Involvement of the baroreceptor reflexes in the changes in blood pressure with sleep and mental arousal. *Hypertension* 1983; **5**: 746–8.

15. Mancia G. Autonomic modulation of the cardiovascular system during sleep. *N Engl J Med* 1993; **328**: 347–9.

16. Lugaresi E, Provini F, Cortelli P. Sleep embodies maximum and minimum levels of autonomic integration. *Clin Auton Res* 2001; **11**: 5–10.

17. Braun AR, Balkin TJ, Wesenstein NJ, et al. Regional cerebral blood flow throughout the sleep-wake cycle. An H20 150 PET study. *Brain* 1997; **120**: 1173–97.

18. Parmeggiani PL, Franzini C. Changes in the activity of hypothalamic units during sleep at different environmental temperatures. *Brain Res* 1971; **29**: 347–50.

19. Buguet AC, Livingstone SD, Reed LD, et al. EEG patterns and body temperatures in man during sleep in arctic winter nights. *Int J Biometeorol* 1976; **20**: 61–9.

20. Coccagna G, Mantovani M, Brignani F, et al. Continuous recording of the pulmonary and systemic arterial pressure during sleep in syndromes of hypersomnia with periodic breathing. *Bull Physiopathol Respir (Nancy)* 1972; **8**: 1159–72.

21. Lugaresi E, Coccagna G, Mantovani M, et al. Hypersomnia with periodic breathing: periodic apneas and alveolar hypoventilation during sleep. *Bull Physiopathol Respir (Nancy)* 1972; **8**: 1103–13.

22. Cortelli P, Pierangeli G, Provini F, et al. Blood pressure rhythms in sleep disorders and dysautonomia. *Ann N Y Acad Sci* 1996; **783**: 204–21.

23. Portaluppi F, Provini F, Cortelli P, et al. Undiagnosed sleep-disordered breathing in male nondippers with essential hypertension. *J Hypertens* 1997; **15**: 1227–33.

24. Portaluppi F, Tiseo R, Smolensky MH, et al. Circadian rhythms and cardiovascular health. *Sleep Med Rev* 2012; **16**: 151–66.

25. Kales A, Bixler EO, Cadieux RJ, et al. Sleep apnoea in a hypertensive population. *Lancet* 1984; **2**: 1005–8.

26. Noda A, Yasuma F, Okada T, et al. Circadian rhythm of autonomic activity in patients with obstructive sleep apnea syndrome. *Clin Cardiol* 1998; **21**: 271–6.

27. Cortelli P, Parchi P, Sforza E, et al. Cardiovascular autonomic dysfunction in normotensive awake subjects with obstructive sleep apnoea syndrome. *Clin Auton Res* 1994; **4**: 57–62.

28. Hargens TA, Guill SG, Zedalis D, et al. Attenuated heart rate recovery following exercise testing in overweight young men with untreated obstructive sleep apnea. *Sleep* 2008; **31**: 104–10.

29. Vanninen E, Tuunainen A, Kansanen M, et al. Cardiac sympathovagal balance during sleep apnea episodes. *Clin Physiol* 1996; **16**: 209–16.

30. Wang W, Tretriluxana S, Redline S, et al. Association of cardiac autonomic function measures with severity of sleep-disordered breathing in a community-based sample. *J Sleep Res* 2008; **17**: 251–62.

31. Méndez MO, Corthout J, Van Huffel S, et al. Automatic screening of obstructive sleep apnea from the ECG based on empirical mode decomposition and wavelet analysis. *Physiol Meas* 2010; **31**: 273–89.

32. Noda A, Nakata S, Koike Y, et al. Continuous positive airway pressure improves daytime baroreflex sensitivity and nitric oxide production in patients with moderate to severe obstructive sleep apnea syndrome. *Hypertens Res* 2007; **30**: 669–76.

33. Baguet JP, Narkiewicz K, Mallion JM. Update on hypertension management: obstructive sleep apnea and hypertension. *J Hypertens* 2006; **24**: 205–8.

34. Friedman O, Logan AG. The price of obstructive sleep apnea-hypopnea: hypertension and other ill effects. *Am J Hypertens* 2009; **22**: 474–83.

35. Watanabe T, Mano T, Iwase S, et al. Enhanced muscle sympathetic nerve activity during sleep apnea in the elderly. *J Auton Nerv Syst* 1992; **37**: 223–6.

36. Donadio V, Liguori R, Vetrugno R, et al. Parallel changes in resting muscle sympathetic nerve activity and blood pressure in a hypertensive OSAS patient demonstrate treatment efficacy. *Clin Auton Res* 2006; **16**: 235–9.

37. Caples SM, Garcia-Touchard A, Somers VK. Sleep-disordered breathing and cardiovascular risk. *Sleep* 2007; **30**: 291–304.

38. Prabhakar NR, Dick TE, Nanduri J, et al. Systemic, cellular and molecular analysis of chemoreflex-mediated sympathoexcitation by chronic intermittent hypoxia. *Exp Physiol* 2007; **92**: 39–44.

39. Brooks D, Horner RL, Kozar LF, et al. Obstructive sleep apnea as a cause of systemic hypertension. Evidence from a canine model. *J Clin Invest* 1997; **99**: 106–9.

40. Narkiewicz KC, Pesek A, Kato M, et al. Baroreflex control of sympathetic nerve activity and heart rate in obstructive sleep apnea. *Hypertension* 1998; **32**: 1039–43.

41. Bonsignore MR, Parati G, Insalaco G, et al. Continuous positive airway pressure treatment improves baroreflex control of heart rate during sleep in severe obstructive sleep apnea syndrome. *Am J Respir Crit Care Med* 2002; **166**: 279–86.

42. Bonsignore MR, Parati G, Insalaco G, et al. Baroreflex control of heart rate during sleep in severe obstructive sleep apnoea: effects of acute CPAP. *Eur Respir J* 2006; **27**: 128–35.

43. Lombardi C, Parati G, Cortelli P, et al. Daytime sleepiness and neural cardiac modulation in sleep-related breathing disorders. *J Sleep Res* 2008; **17**: 263–70.

44. Parati G, Lombardi C, Narkiewicz K. Sleep apnea: epidemiology, pathophysiology, and relation to cardiovascular risk. *Am J Physiol Regul Integr Comp Physiol* 2007; **293**: R1671–83.

45. Prabhakar NR, Kumar GK, Nanduri J. Intermittent hypoxia-mediated plasticity of acute O2 sensing requires altered redox regulation by HIF-1 and HIF-2. *Ann N Y Acad Sci* 2009; **1177**: 162–8.

46. Carlson JT, Hedner JA, Sellgren J, et al. Depressed baroreflex sensitivity in patients with obstructive sleep apnea. *Am J Respir Crit Care Med* 1996; **154**: 1490–6.

47. Parati G, Bonsignore MR, Insalaco G, et al. Autonomic cardiac regulation in obstructive sleep apnea syndrome: evidence from spontaneous baroreflex analysis during sleep. *J Hypertens* 1997; **15**: 1621–6.

48. Kapur VK, Resnick HE, Gottlieb DJ. Sleep disordered breathing and hypertension: does self-reported sleepiness modify the association? *Sleep* 2008; **31**: 1127–32.

49. Barbe F, Mayoralas LR, Duran J, et al. Treatment with continuous positive airway pressure is not effective in patients with sleep apnea but no daytime sleepiness. A randomized, controlled trial. *Ann Intern Med* 2001; **134**: 1015–23.

50. Robinson GV, Smith DM, Langford BA, et al. Continuous positive airway pressure does not reduce blood pressure in nonsleepy hypertensive OSA patients. *Eur Respir J* 2006; **27**: 1229–35.

51. Marrone O, Lombardi C, Parati G. Effects of continuous positive airway pressure therapy on hypertension control in patients

with sleep-related breathing disorders: available evidence and unresolved issues. *J Hypertens* 2010; **28**: 2012–15.

52. Barbe F, Duran-Cantolla J, Capote F, et al. Long-term effect of continuous positive airway pressure in hypertensive patients with sleep apnea. *Am J Respir Crit Care Med* 2010; **181**: 718–26.

53. Vernet C, Redolfi S, Attali V, et al. Residual sleepiness in obstructive sleep apnoea: phenotype and related symptoms. *Eur Respir J* 2011; **38**: 98–105.

54. Vernet C, Redolfi S, Attali V, et al. Why excessive sleepiness may persist in OSA patients receiving adequate CPAP treatment. *Eur Respir J* 2012; **39**: 227–8.

55. Ip MS, Tse HF, Lam B, et al. Endothelial function in obstructive sleep apnea and response to treatment. *Am J Respir Crit Care Med* 2004; **169**: 348–53.

56. Vgontzas AN, Papanicolaou DA, Bixler EO, et al. Sleep apnea and daytime sleepiness and fatigue: relation to visceral obesity, insulin resistance, and hypercytokinemia. *J Clin Endocrinol Metab* 2000; **85**: 1151–8.

57. Boström KB, Hedner J, Melander O, et al. Interaction between the angiotensin-converting enzyme gene insertion/deletion polymorphism and obstructive sleep apnoea as a mechanism for hypertension. *J Hypertens* 2007; **25**: 779–83.

Sleep apnea and hypertension: a clinical perspective

Nishidh Barot and Clete A. Kushida

Sleep apnea as a risk factor for hypertension

Autonomic changes in sleep apnea

In normal sleep there is a significant drop in the mean blood pressure and heart rate, with autonomic tone exhibiting an overall parasympathetic dominance [1]. The reduction in blood pressure is most prominent during slow-wave sleep, which occurs predominantly during the first half of the night. As early as the 1970s, observational studies in patients with obstructive sleep apnea (OSA) demonstrated alterations of normal cardiovascular physiology during sleep [2]. These early studies documented several hemodynamic changes, including cyclic elevations in blood pressure that occur in conjunction with recurrent obstructive apneas. Later studies demonstrated that these hemodynamic changes are driven by changes in autonomic regulation [3]. Obstructive sleep apnea ultimately results in a significant overall increase in sympathetic activity during sleep, which in turn influences heart rate and blood pressure. The increased sympathetic activity appears to be induced through a variety of different mechanisms in OSA, including chemoreflex stimulation (hypoxia, hypercapnea), baroreflexes, pulmonary afferents, the Mueller maneuver, impairment of venous return to the heart, alterations in cardiac output, and possibly the arousal response [3].

One consequence of the autonomic changes is an increase in blood pressure variability, which has repeatedly been demonstrated on ambulatory blood pressure monitoring in patients with OSA [3–5]. During the course of an apnea, there is a progressive increase in sympathetic drive, with maximal sympathetic activity occurring at the end of the apnea. Correspondingly, blood pressure rises progressively, peaking immediately after cessation of the apnea to levels that can reach much higher than baseline; the blood pressure spike has been documented to reach 240/130 mmHg in some subjects [3]. Soon after termination of the apnea and resumption of normal breathing, blood pressure and sympathetic discharge deescalate until the onset of the next obstructive event, at which time they build up progressively again. This repeated cycle of abnormal surges in sympathetic activity and blood pressure throughout sleep results in significant variability in nighttime blood pressure. Additionally, the autonomic instability extends into wakefulness; patients with sleep apnea have been shown to exhibit significantly greater blood pressure variability and sympathetic drive during the daytime as well [4]. The mechanism behind this spillover of autonomic effects into wakefulness is not fully understood, but may be due to an impairment in normal daytime chemoreflex and baroreflex responses from excessive, repetitive stimulation during sleep [4].

Sleep, Stroke, and Cardiovascular Disease, ed. Antonio Culebras. Published by Cambridge University Press. © Cambridge University Press 2013.

The degree of severity of sleep apnea has been shown to correlate with the degree of severity of blood pressure variability. Even patients who have OSA but who do not suffer from clinical hypertension demonstrate greater blood pressure variability, during both the day and the night. Heightened blood pressure variability in sleep apnea may contribute to the development of hypertension and other cardiovascular morbidity. Autonomic instability is considered a risk factor for the future development of hypertension and the first step in its eventual development [6]. In patients who suffer from hypertension, those who demonstrate greater blood pressure variability also have greater cardiovascular morbidity, independent of the degree of hypertension [4].

Nondipping, nocturnal hypertension, and morning hypertension

Blood pressure values normally drop by around 10%–20% during sleep compared to daytime values, a phenomenon known as dipping [1]. Nondipping, defined as less than a 10% drop in blood pressure during the night, is common in sleep apnea, and increases in prevalence as the severity of sleep apnea increases [7]. In 2008, Hla et al. [7] performed an analysis of blood pressure trends in a sample of patients from the Wisconsin Sleep Cohort Study. The study included 328 patients, followed longitudinally for several years, and revealed that patients with sleep apnea were more likely to develop a nondipping pattern to systolic blood pressure during the night. The likelihood of nondipping increased with increasing severity of sleep apnea. Furthermore, the association between OSA and nondipping persisted after accounting for BMI, age, gender, medications, and other potential confounding factors.

Other studies have demonstrated an overall increase in nighttime and morning blood pressure measurements in patients with sleep apnea [5]. Several studies have demonstrated an increase in the 24-hour mean arterial blood pressure in sleep apnea, but ambulatory blood pressure monitoring has shown that the greatest period of elevation in OSA occurs during the night. Here again there appears to be a direct relationship between severity of sleep apnea and severity of nocturnal blood pressure elevation. More severe cases of sleep apnea often demonstrate nocturnal hypertension, which remains refractory to medications. Studies that have evaluated the nocturnal blood pressure changes in sleep apnea suggest a causal role of sleep apnea in nondipping of blood pressure, nocturnal hypertension, and elevation of morning blood pressures [5,7].

These well-demonstrated nocturnal cardiovascular effects of OSA have important implications, independent of any effects on cardiovascular parameters that also occur during the day. Studies in hypertensive populations to date suggest that nondipping during the night, heightened blood pressure variability during the night, and nocturnal hypertension all predict future risk for cardiovascular morbidity and mortality, and are better prognostic factors than daytime hypertension [4,7,8]. One prospective study measured ambulatory blood pressure in 1332 Japanese adults over the age of forty years [8]. When comparing the prognostic value of daytime versus nighttime blood pressure measurements, only the nighttime blood pressure values significantly predicted future cardiovascular mortality over a follow-up period of over 10 years.

Daytime hypertension

In addition to the nocturnal effects of sleep apnea on blood pressure, there also appears to be an association between sleep apnea and daytime hypertension, although this is controversial due to mixed results in the literature [9]. In 2000, Nieto et al. [10] performed a cross-sectional analysis of data on 6132 middle-aged and older subjects enrolled in the multicenter Sleep Heart Health Study, all of whom had daytime blood pressure measurements and unattended polysomnography in their homes. An association was discovered between increasing severity of OSA and an increase in both systolic and diastolic blood pressures; the association was present in both genders and all ethnicities, and persisted after correction for potential confounders such as BMI. Another large analysis in 2000, performed by Peppard et al. [11], followed 709 subjects from the Wisconsin Sleep Cohort Study for four years after baseline overnight polysomnography to determine the association between sleep-disordered breathing (SDB) and daytime hypertension. A dose–response relationship between the severity of SDB at baseline and the likelihood of having hypertension four years later was found.

Data from these and other large-scale population studies clearly demonstrate a dose-dependent relationship between OSA and hypertension; however, whether OSA plays an independent role in daytime systemic hypertension is a matter of debate. Some have attributed the observed association between OSA and hypertension to confounding variables, in particular obesity, which is more common in patients with OSA [12]. There is some evidence to suggest that sleep apnea may play a greater role in the development of hypertension in a specific subset of hypertensive patients. This includes those with resistant hypertension, defined as suboptimal control of blood pressure despite adequate doses of more than two antihypertensives [13,14]. Obstructive sleep apnea may also play a greater role in those hypertensives who exhibit nondipping of blood pressures at night [15,16]. Some evidence suggests that OSA plays a greater contributory role in hypertension in the younger and middle-aged population, compared to the elderly [10,17]. There is also evidence to suggest that the severity of OSA influences the effect on blood pressure, with a higher apnea/hypopnea index (AHI) and greater oxygen desaturations showing stronger associations with hypertension [10].

Studies that have demonstrated a reduction in daytime blood pressure after OSA treatment have also provided evidence of a contributory role of sleep apnea in hypertension. Although there are some conflicting data, most interventional trials suggest that treatment of OSA lowers blood pressure in hypertensive patients [18–34]. Some studies have also shown that treatment of sleep apnea can prevent the development of overt hypertension in those who have borderline high blood pressures. One study in patients with severe OSA demonstrated a significant reduction in prehypertension and masked hypertension [18]. Another small study in patients with upper airway resistance syndrome, a form of sleep apnea without significant oxygen desaturations, demonstrated that borderline hypertension could be brought under control with continuous positive airway pressure (CPAP) treatment [19]. The effects of sleep apnea treatment on hypertension are discussed in further detail later in this chapter and in Chapter 10.

Other evidence of a causal role of OSA in daytime hypertension comes from experiments in animals. In one study, recurrent episodes of upper airway occlusion with oxygen desaturations were introduced during sleep in several dogs [35]. Daytime hypertension ensued within four weeks. Within three weeks of discontinuation of the intervention, daytime blood pressures had returned to normal. Furthermore, when repetitive electroencephalographic (EEG) arousals from sleep without airway occlusion (and hypoxia) were introduced, daytime blood pressure did not rise, suggesting that other factors, such as repetitive arousals, were not the cause of the hypertension.

Obesity, sleep apnea, and hypertension

Obesity, sleep apnea, and hypertension frequently coexist [36]. Obesity is considered a strong risk factor for both hypertension and sleep apnea. Although the exact mechanism by which obesity causes hypertension is not known, pathophysiological observations in obesity suggest various possible mechanisms. These include the associations between obesity and the following: increased sympathetic drive, stimulation of the renin–angiotensin system, inflammation, oxidative stress, insulin resistance, hyperleptinemia with leptin resistance, and autonomic derangement. Interestingly, many similar associations are found in sleep apnea [36]. What is even more noteworthy is the observation that when obese patients are separated into those with and those without sleep apnea, several of the typical obesity-associated physiological changes significantly attenuate in those without sleep apnea. For example, in one study comparing differences in sympathetic activity between obese patients with OSA, obese patients without OSA, and non-obese patients, those obese patients who did not have sleep apnea showed no significant difference in measures of sympathetic activity when compared to non-obese patients; however, the obese patients with comorbid sleep apnea showed significantly higher measures of sympathetic activity than either of the other two groups [37]. In addition, plasma levels of leptin, a hormone the functions of which include appetite and blood pressure control, are known to be elevated in obese patients. Studies have shown that plasma levels of leptin are elevated to a greater degree in obese patients with sleep apnea compared to BMI-matched obese patients who do not have OSA, suggesting a greater degree of hyperleptinemia and leptin resistance in OSA [38].

Some argue that obesity is the primary explanation for the apparent association between sleep apnea and hypertension [12,39]. In contrast, others have speculated that because OSA was not accounted for in epidemiological studies of obesity and hypertension, it should be considered as a candidate mechanism by which obesity is linked to hypertension and other cardiovascular effects that have traditionally been attributed to obesity itself [36,40]. Adding uncertainty to causal determination is evidence that suggests that the relationship between obesity and OSA is not unidirectional. Obesity has been a well-known risk factor for OSA, but current observations suggest that OSA can actually contribute to obesity through a variety of putative mechanisms [36]. Indeed, in obese patients who suffer from OSA, CPAP treatment has been demonstrated to reduce visceral fat accumulation [41]. Obese patients with untreated OSA can therefore develop a "vicious cycle" of mutually worsening comorbidities, which only complicates attempts to separate the independent effects of each condition [36]. At this point, it is difficult to tease apart the relative contributions of OSA and obesity to hypertension and other cardiovascular complications. Definitive quantifications of the independent effect of sleep apnea on hypertension in obese patients are hard to ascertain. What appears certain is that, at the very least, OSA exasperates several pathophysiological abnormalities that are thought to lead eventually to hypertension in obese patients, and therefore contribute to obesity-related cardiovascular morbidity.

Predictors of sleep apnea in hypertension

Hypertensive populations at risk

Patients with OSA are at significant risk of developing hypertension. Because of various methodological reasons, estimates of the prevalence of hypertension in those with OSA vary significantly between different studies; however, in all reports the risk for hypertension is uniformly greater than in those persons without sleep apnea, and several estimates suggest that more than 50% of patients with OSA suffer from hypertension [41]. The risk of hypertension in OSA correlates with the severity of OSA, as more severe OSA shows a greater prevalence of hypertension. In the 2000 Sleep Heart Health analysis performed by Nieto et al. [10], the unadjusted odds ratio for hypertension in the highest AHI category (AHI >30 events/h), compared to the lowest AHI category (AHI <1.5 events/h), was 2.27. Likewise, patients with hypertension are more likely to suffer from underlying OSA. Estimates of the prevalence of OSA in hypertension also vary, with several studies showing that more than 30% of hypertensive patients suffer from OSA [17,42,43].

Certain hypertensive populations are at greater risk for OSA; several subgroups of hypertensive patients, including some mentioned earlier in the chapter, demonstrate a stronger correlation between sleep apnea and hypertension. Hypertensive patients who are of a younger age, and those who suffer from obesity, metabolic syndrome, resistant hypertension, or non-dipping of blood pressures during sleep are more likely to suffer from OSA [17,39,44–52]. Although the prevalence of OSA increases with age, younger patients with OSA may be more prone to having cardiovascular consequences, including hypertension. Several studies suggest that the association between OSA and hypertension is more robust in the non-elderly [17,44]. As mentioned earlier, obesity, OSA, and hypertension often coexist; not surprisingly, those hypertensive patients who are obese are more likely to have OSA [39,45].

Even more impressive is the strength of the association between metabolic syndrome and OSA. The conditions that collectively comprise metabolic syndrome, namely hypertension, dyslipidemia, truncal obesity, and insulin resistance, have each been associated with sleep apnea; the clustering together of these conditions in metabolic syndrome proves to be a fairly sensitive and specific indicator for the risk of OSA [46]. One study has demonstrated metabolic syndrome to have a sensitivity and specificity for OSA of 86% and 85%, respectively, with positive and negative predictive values for OSA of 87% and 82%, respectively [47]. Findings such as these have prompted some to use the term "syndrome Z," which adds sleep apnea to the cardinal features of metabolic syndrome [48,49]. That OSA can contribute to the development of metabolic syndrome and its components is supported by recent evidence showing improvement of metabolic abnormalities and hypertension in metabolic syndrome after initiation of CPAP treatment [46].

Another population at high risk for OSA consists of those with resistant hypertension. The prevalence of OSA in resistant hypertension is exceedingly high; in one study, those with resistant hypertension were more than 2.5 times more likely than controlled hypertensives to meet criteria for high risk for OSA as measured by the apnea risk evaluation system (ARES) questionnaire [50]. In another study around 85% of patients with resistant hypertension were found to have OSA [51]. In addition, a study that evaluated consecutive patients with resistant hypertension for established secondary causes revealed that sleep apnea was by far the most common secondary cause, more common than all other secondary causes combined, with 64% of patients found to have moderate to severe OSA. The next most common cause, primary aldosteronism, was found in only 5.6% of patients [13]. Not only is OSA extremely common in resistant hypertension, but evidence suggests that it contributes more to the development of hypertension in this subgroup of patients. Continuous positive airway pressure is more effective at lowering blood pressure in OSA patients with resistant hypertension compared to OSA patients with controlled hypertension; consequently, CPAP treatment is more likely to permit adjustments of antihypertensive medication in this subgroup as well [52].

Nondipping on ambulatory blood pressure monitoring may identify another high risk group of hypertensive patients. It has been well documented that those with OSA are more likely to have nondipping of blood pressure, and that CPAP treatment of sleep apnea can restore the normal dipping pattern; however, screening studies among nondippers to determine the prevalence of OSA in that population have been scant [7,16]. In one small study, 10 out of 11 nondippers were found to have sleep apnea [16]. Studies of patients who have OSA suggest that nondippers comprise a relatively small percentage of hypertensive patients and of OSA patients; however, the presence of nondipping, although not a sensitive method for OSA detection, does appear to have a high specificity for OSA. Obstructive sleep apnea should, therefore, be suspected in all hypertensive patients who demonstrate non-dipping of blood pressures during sleep [16].

Screening for obstructive sleep apnea in hypertensive patients

The 2011 the American College of Cardiology Foundation and American Heart Association (ACCF/AHA) Expert Consensus Document on Hypertension in the Elderly recognizes OSA as a secondary cause of hypertension. It acknowledges that OSA appears to have a stronger association with hypertension in adults younger than 60 years of age, deserving special consideration in this population [53]. The 2003 seventh report of the Joint National Committee (JNC) on Prevention, Detection, Evaluation, and Treatment of High Blood Pressure also recognizes sleep apnea as an identifiable cause of hypertension that needs to be considered during clinical evaluation of the hypertensive patient [54]. Because obesity often coexists, the JNC recommends a high index of suspicion for OSA in any hypertensive patient with a BMI of >27. The JNC seventh report goes on to recommend thorough questioning in these patients about OSA-related symptoms, including snoring, witnessed apneas or irregular breathing, morning fatigue, and restless sleeping. Questioning of bed partners is specifically recommended as well, as patients themselves are often unaware of sleep-related symptoms such as snoring and other irregularities of breathing [54]. All patients in whom OSA is clinically suspected are recommended to undergo overnight polysomnography with oximetry.

Different screening questionnaires have been developed and tested in attempts to identify patients at high risk for OSA. The Epworth sleepiness scale (ESS) is probably the most commonly used screening tool in the general population for sleep disorders (including sleep apnea), but it has been demonstrated to have poor sensitivity in the screening of OSA [55]. In one study, the ESS was used as a screening tool in a high-risk population of patients with both hypertension and obesity; it identified 10% to have sleep apnea [39]. The significantly higher prevalence of OSA in this population demonstrated in other studies suggests the need for more sensitive methods of screening in hypertension [47]. Many other screening questionnaires incorporate hypertension as one of the components to help determine high risk. The Berlin questionnaire incorporates three different categories, including symptoms during sleep (snoring), daytime symptoms (sleepiness), and medical comorbidities (hypertension, obesity), to stratify patients into low-risk and high-risk groups. In one study by Netzer et al. [56], 744 subjects from the general population completed the Berlin questionnaire, of whom 100 patients taken from both the high- and low-risk groups underwent confirmatory ambulatory polysomnography. Those who were high-risk in at least two of the three categories were classified as overall high-risk, while those who were high-risk in fewer than two categories were classified as overall low-risk individuals. Using this method, the Berlin questionnaire demonstrated a fairly high sensitivity at 86% in predicting those with a respiratory disturbance index

(RDI) of >5. The specificity of the questionnaire in this sample of community-dwelling adults was about 77%, and the positive predictive value was 89%. Risk grouping by combining the three different categories predicted those with OSA better than did any one category alone.

The STOP questionnaire is another screening tool that incorporates hypertension to help determine high risk [55,57]. It consists of four components (STOP): snoring, tiredness, observed apneas, and blood pressure. A variation of the STOP questionnaire, called the STOP-BANG questionnaire, adds four more components (BANG): BMI, age, neck circumference, and gender, resulting in even greater screening sensitivity for OSA. In one analysis, the STOP-BANG questionnaire was demonstrated to have a sensitivity of 87.0% for detecting moderate to severe OSA, although specificity was only 43.3% [55]. In a further analysis it was found to have 100% sensitivity for the detection of severe OSA, defined as an AHI of >30 events/h on overnight in-laboratory polysomnography [57]. Another screening measure, the four-variable screening tool, determines risk by calculating a score based on BMI, gender, blood pressure, and snoring. It has been demonstrated to be a more specific but less sensitive method of screening for OSA when compared to the STOP-BANG questionnaire [55]. Some other screening questionnaires, such as the sleep apnea sleep disorders questionnaire (SA-SDQ), also include hypertension as a criterion to determine high risk for OSA [58].

A comprehensive meta-analysis of the different screening tools for OSA performed in 2009 by Ramachandran and Josephs [59] demonstrated that although some may be helpful, no single questionnaire is ideal, especially because of unacceptably high false-negative rates for less severe cases of OSA. Comparisons of the available questionnaires that have been used and studied suggest that the Berlin questionnaire and the STOP-BANG questionnaires appear to be the most accurate in predicting risk of OSA, particularly severe OSA; both questionnaires use hypertension as a criterion to help determine high risk [58–60]. It should be noted that most screening tests have not been tested specifically in purely hypertensive populations. False-negative results would be particularly problematic in this group, which already has a higher pretest probability for sleep apnea.

Specific medical comorbidities alluded to earlier should raise the index of suspicion for possible sleep apnea in hypertensive patients. In several cases, the presence of a high-risk medical comorbidity may be of greater predictive value than any questionnaire or other screening method. One study in 2010 by Drager et al [47] compared different variables, including age, gender, snoring, daytime sleepiness, obesity, resistant hypertension, metabolic syndrome, and the Berlin questionnaire, to predict OSA in a group of 99 hypertensive patients. All patients had standard overnight polysomnography performed. Obstructive sleep apnea was defined as an AHI of >5 events/h. Obesity had reasonable specificity at 75%, but had a lower sensitivity at only 58%, as many non-obese hypertensive patients also have sleep apnea [47]. The presence of resistant hypertension was a highly specific predictor of OSA at 91%; however, sensitivity for detecting OSA was even lower than obesity at 41%. Both the Berlin questionnaire and patient age (between 40 and 70 years) had greater than 90% sensitivity, although both were below 60% in specificity. Of all the variables that were under consideration in the study, metabolic syndrome was the most accurate predictor of sleep apnea, demonstrating both high sensitivity and specificity at 86% and 85%, respectively. Other studies have also shown a high positive predictive value of metabolic syndrome for OSA, leading some to argue for diagnostic polysomnography in all patients with metabolic syndrome, regardless of sleep symptomatology [48]. Certainly, because of the strong association between the two, clinicians should have a very low threshold to refer for sleep evaluation in any hypertensive patients with metabolic syndrome.

Several of the different screening methods and predictors for OSA could be utilized easily in clinical practice to identify hypertensive patients who are at particularly high risk for sleep apnea. Use of a simple questionnaire, such as the Berlin questionnaire or STOP-BANG questionnaire, could prove to be a fairly easy method for primary care physicians, cardiologists, or nephrologists to identify a large pool of higher-risk hypertensive patients who should undergo further sleep evaluation. Recognition of highly specific predictors of sleep apnea in a hypertensive patient's medical history can facilitate appropriate further sleep work-up. These predictors include resistant hypertension, metabolic syndrome, and those with a history of comparatively high nocturnal blood pressures (nondippers) and/or morning blood pressures. Because of a very high pretest probability for OSA, these patients could bypass other simple screening considerations and proceed directly toward further sleep evaluation. In summary, the index of suspicion for OSA should be high for any hypertensive patient who has suggestive symptoms (snoring, witnessed apneas, unrefreshing sleep) [54] or who falls into any other high-risk populations (younger patients, those with nocturnal or morning hypertension, obesity, metabolic syndrome, resistant hypertension) [16,20,47]. A careful medical history and, if necessary, appropriate ancillary questionnaires can be simple, helpful screening methods to identify high-risk patients who require formal sleep evaluation.

Effects of obstructive sleep apnea treatment on hypertension

Continuous positive airway pressure

Almost all studies investigating the treatment of OSA have evaluated the effect of CPAP, the gold standard of treatment for OSA. Although there is some discordance in the findings among various studies, most studies demonstrate some form of an effect on blood pressure in hypertensive patients with OSA [18–34]. Several studies have also demonstrated effects of CPAP on coexisting autonomic abnormalities in OSA, which are thought to play an etiological role in the development of hypertension. For example, CPAP has been demonstrated to reduce circulating catecholamine levels [21,22] and reduce variability in blood pressure while both asleep and awake [23]. Continuous positive airway pressure has also been demonstrated to improve 48-hour circadian blood pressure profiles in hypertensive patients with OSA [24].

Two different meta-analyses of randomized trials evaluating the impact of CPAP on blood pressure in OSA patients revealed a small but significant reduction in mean arterial blood pressure, on the order of around 2 mm Hg [25,26]. Such an overall effect of CPAP treatment may on the surface appear fairly miniscule. Indeed, when CPAP was compared to a typical antihypertensive medication, the medication caused a reduction in blood pressure that was approximately four times greater than that of CPAP [27]. However, interpretation of the cardiovascular effects of CPAP requires recognition of several factors. One important factor to consider is that, over long periods of time, small differences in blood pressure can translate into large differences in cardiovascular outcomes. A large review of several prospective studies demonstrated that over about 10 years, a 5 mmHg lower diastolic blood pressure was associated with at least 34% lower risk for stroke and 21% lower risk for coronary artery disease [28].

Another important factor to consider is that the effect of CPAP on blood pressure may be greater in select populations. The reported effects of CPAP on blood pressure in different interventional trials are drawn from a heterogeneous population of patients, including those with milder OSA, fewer symptoms, varying levels of CPAP compliance, and normal baseline blood pressure; therefore, the overall pooled results may underestimate the impact of treatment in select populations. Several studies have demonstrated a greater degree of blood pressure reduction from CPAP in patients with more severe baseline OSA, more severe baseline hypertension, a nocturnal nondipping pattern to blood pressures, greater levels of pretreatment daytime sleepiness, and better CPAP compliance [15,18,22,28–32,34,52]. One of the 2007 meta-analyses [25] concluded that CPAP has a greater effect on blood pressure in those with more severe OSA, with a decrease in 24-hour mean arterial blood pressure (MAP) by 0.89 mmHg per every 10-point increase in the original AHI. A 2011 trial examined the effect of CPAP only in patients with severe OSA, with the average AHI around 56, and demonstrated an effect of CPAP on systolic blood pressure of 5 mmHg [18]. Another study of the long-term effects of CPAP evaluated changes in blood pressure in 55 OSA patients with hypertension after 24 months of CPAP usage. The study revealed greater reductions in blood pressure in those with greater CPAP compliance; those in whom average CPAP compliance was greater than 5.3 hours per night had a decrease in 24-hour MAP of 5.3 mmHg [28]. Both 2007 meta-analyses also confirmed that the degree that CPAP reduced blood pressure was proportionate to CPAP compliance [25,26]. In one of the meta-analyses, every one hour increase in CPAP usage led to a reduction in blood pressure by 1.39 mmHg [25]. (Further discussion of this topic is found in Chapter 10.)

Oral appliance and surgical treatment

Far fewer studies have evaluated the effect of other treatments on blood pressure for sleep apnea. Very few randomized controlled trials have evaluated the effect of oral appliance (OA) therapy or surgical treatments for OSA on blood pressure. In one randomized, controlled crossover trial, 61 patients with OSA underwent 24-hour ambulatory blood pressure monitoring after four weeks of treatment with a mandibular advancement splint or a control oral appliance [62]. Those in the treatment arm of the study demonstrated a reduction in awake systolic blood pressures (SBP) and diastolic blood pressures (DBP) compared to a placebo, although there was no significant difference in blood pressures while asleep. In another prospective, nonrandomized study, 11 adults with both OSA and hypertension underwent oral appliance treatment; ambulatory blood pressure measurements were taken over a 20-hour period before and after a several-month titration to a therapeutic jaw position [63]. After titration, patients demonstrated reductions in SBP, DBP, and MAP during the night, as well as reductions in DBP and MAP over the entire 20-hour period.

Studies of the effects on blood pressure from surgical treatment of OSA have occurred mostly in children. Children who suffer from OSA are more likely to exhibit abnormally increased blood pressures during wakefulness and sleep [64,65]. Those children with both OSA and hypertension, who are adequately treated for OSA by adenotonsillectomy, experience a long-term improvement in blood pressure [64,66]. The effect of surgery on blood pressure appears directly related to the effectiveness of the surgery on treating OSA. One study evaluated the long-term effect of adenotonsillectomy on OSA and blood pressure; those children with recurrence of OSA one year after surgery were more likely to experience recurrence of elevation in systolic blood pressures as well [64].

Treatment of hyperaldosteronism and peripheral edema

Over the past few years several studies have suggested that peripheral edema may contribute to the pathophysiology of sleep apnea in certain hypertensive OSA patients. In OSA patients with peripheral edema, excess extracellular fluid, which normally falls to the dependent areas of the legs during the day, can undergo rostral displacement while recumbent during sleep. The pharyngeal tissues in these patients become more edematous during the sleep period, resulting in narrowing of the pharyngeal walls, which in turn contributes to obstruction of the upper airway [67]. Several studies in heart failure patients have demonstrated that the degree of severity of OSA depends upon the amount of rostral fluid shift that occurs overnight, as measured by the overnight decrease in calf circumference and increase in neck circumference [67,68]. One study evaluated the effect of three days of inpatient diuretic treatment on 15 patients with diastolic heart failure and coexisting hypertension and severe OSA [67]. In addition to reducing body weight and blood pressure, treatment with diuretics also increased the patency of the upper airway and reduced the severity of OSA. In one study of CPAP treatment for patients with systolic heart failure and OSA, CPAP was demonstrated to prevent the nocturnal increase in neck circumference, suggesting a different, novel mechanism by which CPAP may treat OSA in these patients [68].

A few studies suggest that upper airway edema may also contribute to the etiology of OSA in patients with drug-resistant hypertension [69,70]. The severity of OSA in patients with resistant hypertension has been demonstrated to be proportionate to the degree of rostral fluid shift that occurs overnight [69]. Patients with resistant hypertension often have hyperaldosteronism, and aldosterone status has been shown to correlate with the severity of OSA in patients with resistant hypertension, presumably because of upper airway edema from excessive salt and fluid retention. In one study of 109 patients with resistant hypertension, 28% were found to have hyperaldosteronism and 77% were found to have OSA [70]. While the majority of OSA patients had normal aldosterone status, those with hyperaldosteronism had more severe OSA, and the amount of aldosterone excess predicted OSA severity. These findings further suggest that aldosterone status and fluid retention partly contribute to the pathophysiology of OSA in some patients, and may need to be considered in the treatment strategy of patients who have heart failure or resistant hypertension. More studies exploring the relationship of peripheral edema and aldosterone status in OSA are necessary, however, before broader treatment recommendations can be made.

Special considerations

Pregnancy

Gestational hypertension develops in about 10% of all pregnancies, and about 12%–22% of pregnancies are complicated by the presence of hypertension [71,72]. Snoring, witnessed apneas, daytime sleepiness, and other symptoms of sleep apnea are more common in women during pregnancy, and are independently associated with an increased likelihood of hypertension [73,74]. In one survey of over 500 pregnant women, snoring was reported every day during the last week of pregnancy in 23% of women, as compared to 4% of the same women prior to pregnancy. Women who consistently snored were more than twice as likely, during pregnancy, to develop hypertension, preeclampsia, and growth retardation of the fetus [73]. In a smaller study of pregnant women, 17 women with gestational hypertension were compared to 33 women without hypertension, and overnight polysomnography was performed to evaluate for the presence of OSA [71]. Those with gestational hypertension were much more likely to have OSA, with an adjusted odds ratio of 7.5. A 2011 study of Taiwanese women compared 791 women who had polysomnographically diagnosed OSA to 3955 women without OSA [75]. Pregnant women with OSA demonstrated an increased risk for having preterm, small-for-gestational-age, and low-birth weight infants, and had a higher rate of preeclampsia and cesarean sections. Some have hypothesized that the edema that accompanies preeclampsia may itself contribute to development of OSA by causing upper airway obstruction, similar to the mechanisms discussed earlier [74].

Support for an etiological role of OSA in gestational hypertension comes from data to suggest that treatment of sleep apnea in pregnancy can improve cardiovascular outcomes. In one small study, sixteen non-obese women with hypertension and symptoms of sleep apnea during pregnancy were randomized to receive either pharmacological treatment alone or pharmacological treatment plus CPAP [72]. Women in the CPAP group had better controlled blood pressure and required significantly lower doses of antihypertensive medication during pregnancy. The CPAP-treated women also delivered infants with higher APGAR scores at one minute after delivery when compared to those with pharmacological treatment alone. Collectively, the data from different studies in pregnant women suggest that OSA may cause gestational hypertension and other associated complications during pregnancy.

Pediatrics

Children with sleep apnea are more likely to have abnormal blood pressures than those without OSA. A 2011 study involving 105 children with OSA demonstrated a nocturnal blood pressure elevation of 10–15 mmHg on ambulatory blood pressure monitoring. Interestingly, the blood pressure elevation was independent of the severity of OSA [65]. Another study of 140 children with sleep apnea demonstrated that even the mildest cases in children are associated with some abnormalities of blood pressure on 24-hour ambulatory monitoring [76]. Children with OSA were also found to have signs of cardiac remodeling on echocardiography, proportionate to the degree of hypertension. In another study that was alluded to earlier, children with OSA were monitored for one year after adenotonsillectomy (64). Diastolic blood pressures improved after six months in all children. After one year, the AHI predicted systolic and diastolic blood pressures improved, even after accounting for BMI, ethnicity, and other confounding variables. The rate of increase in BMI, African–American ethnicity, and overall weight status were also predictors of hypertension, as well as of recurrence of SDB.

Pulmonary hypertension

Pulmonary hypertension (PHT), defined as a pulmonary artery pressure of >20 mmHg, is common in OSA. About 20%–40% of OSA patients have PHT without having any other known cardiopulmonary source for PHT [77]. Pulmonary hypertension secondary to OSA is typically mild, although severe PHT has been observed in OSA as well [78]. Higher BMI, higher AHI, a greater degree of nocturnal oxygen desaturation, and the presence of daytime hypoxia/hypercapnea have all been demonstrated to be predictors for both the presence and severity of PHT in OSA patients [78,79].

Obesity hypoventilation syndrome (OHS) is defined by the presence of SDB, obesity (BMI >30), and alveolar hypoventilation as evidenced by daytime hypercapnia ($paCO_2$ >45 mmHg) and hypoxia (paO_2 <70 mmHg) occurring in the absence of other pulmonary or neuromuscular disease [80,81]. The vast majority (90%) of those with OHS have OSA as the form of SDB, with the remainder (10%) suffering from sleep hypoventilation, where hypoxia and hypercapnia occur without any identifiable obstructive apneas or hypopneas [81]. Around 10%–20% of those with OSA have coexisting OHS, and its prevalence in OSA increases with increases in BMI [81]. Obesity hypoventilation syndrome encompasses many of the high-risk attributes for OSA-related pulmonary hypertension. Not surprisingly, OHS patients constitute a subgroup of OSA patients who are at greater risk for pulmonary hypertension, with about 50% of OHS patients suffering from PHT [82].

That SDB can contribute to PHT is confirmed by a demonstrated reduction in pulmonary artery pressures after adequate treatment of OSA. Several studies have demonstrated an improvement in pulmonary artery pressures after beginning CPAP treatment for OSA [79,82,83]. In one study of 29 patients with OSA and no other pulmonary disorders, six were found to have PHT on echocardiography [79]. After six months of treatment with CPAP, all 29 patients demonstrated a reduction in pulmonary artery pressures. Those with mild pulmonary hypertension had an average reduction in pulmonary artery pressure of 6.1 mmHg; however, even those without PHT showed a reduction in pulmonary artery pressures of an average of 3.4 mmHg. Importantly, there was no significant change in BMI during the course of the study.

Pediatric studies have demonstrated that children with significant adenotonsillar hypertrophy, in addition to exhibiting greater symptoms of OSA, are more likely to have pulmonary hypertension and right ventricular impairment, as measured by Doppler echocardiography [84,85]. Both pulmonary hypertension and right ventricular performance improve significantly after adenotonsillectomy treatment in these children. In one study of 52 children with adenotonsillar hypertrophy, the mean pulmonary artery pressure decreased from 23 mmHg preoperatively to 17 mmHg postoperatively [84]. The majority (18 out of 27) of those who met the criteria for PHT preoperatively had a decrease in pulmonary artery pressures to within the normal range after surgery. In combination with the CPAP treatment data in adults with OSA and PHT, the data regarding surgical treatment of OSA strongly support a causal role of SDB in the development of PHT.

Conclusion

There is a growing body of convincing evidence that demonstrates that OSA is an independent risk factor for hypertension. Obstructive sleep apnea contributes more greatly to hypertension in certain subgroups of hypertensive patients, including younger patients, and those with more severe OSA, more daytime sleepiness, more severe hypertension, and nondipping of blood pressures. More aggressive screening for OSA is necessary in hypertensive patients; simple screening methods include questioning about OSA symptoms, the use of questionnaires, and recognition of certain hypertensive populations that are at particularly high risk for OSA. Treatments for OSA, of which CPAP is the best studied, have been demonstrated to reduce blood pressure in OSA patients. The amount of reduction in blood pressure from OSA treatment depends upon several factors, but even small reductions in blood pressure can translate into significant improvement in long-term clinical outcomes. More studies are necessary to further elucidate pathogenetic mechanisms by which OSA causes hypertension and to determine the magnitude of the effect of OSA and its treatments on blood pressure.

References

1. Coccagna G, Mantovani M, Brignani F, et al. Laboratory note. Arterial pressure changes during spontaneous sleep in man. *Electroencephalogr Clin Neurophysiol* 1971; **31**: 277–81.

2. Tilkian AG, Guilleminault C, Schroeder JS, et al. Hemodynamics in sleep-induced apnea. Studies during wakefulness and sleep. *Ann Intern Med* 1976; **85**: 714–19.

3. Somers VK, Dyken ME, Clary MP, et al. Sympathetic neural mechanisms in obstructive sleep apnea. *J Clin Invest* 1995; **96**: 1897–904.

4. Narkiewicz K, Montano N, Cogliati C, et al. Altered cardiovascular variability in obstructive sleep apnea. *Circulation* 1998; **98**: 1071–7.

5. Nagata K, Osada N, Shimazaki M, et al. Diurnal blood pressure variation in patients with sleep apnea syndrome. *Hypertens Res* 2008; **31**: 185–91.

6. Singh JP, Larson MG, Tsuji H, et al. Reduced heart rate variability and new-onset hypertension: insights into pathogenesis of hypertension: the Framingham Heart Study. *Hypertension* 1998; **32**: 293–7.

7. Hla KM, Young T, Finn L, et al. Longitudinal association of sleep-disordered breathing and nondipping of nocturnal blood pressure in the Wisconsin Sleep Cohort Study. *Sleep* 2008; **31**: 795–800.

8. Kikuya M, Ohkubo T, Asayama K, et al. Ambulatory blood pressure and 10-year risk of cardiovascular and noncardiovascular mortality: the Ohasama study. *Hypertension* 2005; **45**: 240–5.

9. Kushida CA, Littner MR, Morgenthaler T, et al. Practice parameters for the indications for polysomnography and related procedures: an update for 2005. *Sleep* 2005; **28**: 499–521.

10. Nieto FJ, Young TB, Lind BK, et al. Association of sleep-disordered breathing, sleep apnea, and hypertension in a large community-based study. Sleep Heart Health Study. *JAMA* 2000; **283**: 1829–36.

11. Peppard PE, Young T, Palta M, et al. Prospective study of the association between sleep-disordered breathing and hypertension. *N Engl J Med* 2000; **342**: 1378–84.

12. Cano-Pumarega I, Durán-Cantolla J, Aizpuru F, et al. Obstructive sleep apnea and systemic hypertension: longitudinal study in the general population: the Vitoria Sleep Cohort. *Am J Respir Crit Care Med* 2011; **184**: 1299–304.

13. Pedrosa RP, Drager LF, Gonzaga CC, et al. Obstructive sleep apnea: the most common secondary cause of hypertension associated with resistant hypertension. *Hypertension* 2011; **58**: 811–17.

14. Logan AG, Perlikowski SM, Mente A, et al. High prevalence of unrecognized sleep apnoea in drug-resistant hypertension. *J Hypertens* 2001; **19**: 2271–7.

15. Lozano L, Tovar JL, Sampol G, et al. Continuous positive airway pressure treatment in sleep apnea patients with resistant hypertension: a randomized, controlled trial. *J Hypertens* 2010; **28**: 2161–8.

16. Portaluppi F, Provini F, Cortelli P, et al. Undiagnosed sleep-disordered breathing among male nondippers with essential hypertension. *J Hypertens* 1997; **15**: 1227–33.

17. Sjöström C, Lindberg E, Elmasry A, et al. Prevalence of sleep apnoea and snoring in hypertensive men: a population based study. *Thorax* 2002; **57**: 602–7.

18. Drager LF, Pedrosa RP, Diniz PM, et al. The effects of continuous positive airway pressure on prehypertension and masked hypertension in men with severe obstructive sleep apnea. *Hypertension* 2011; **57**: 549–55.

19. Guilleminault C, Stoohs R, Shiomi T, et al. Upper airway resistance syndrome, nocturnal blood pressure monitoring, and borderline hypertension. *Chest* 1996; **109**: 901–8.

20. Budhiraja R, Quan SF. When is CPAP an antihypertensive in sleep apnea patients? *J Clin Sleep Med* 2009; **5**: 108–9.

21. Jennum P, Wildschiødtz G, Christensen NJ, et al. Blood pressure, catecholamines, and pancreatic polypeptide in obstructive sleep apnea with and without nasal continuous positive airway pressure (nCPAP) treatment. *Am J Hypertens* 1989; **2**: 847–52.

22. Heitmann J, Ehlenz K, Penzel T, et al. Sympathetic activity is reduced by nCPAP in hypertensive obstructive sleep apnoea patients. *Eur Respir J* 2004; **23**: 255–62.

23. Mayer J, Becker H, Brandenburg U, et al. Blood pressure and sleep apnea: results of long-term nasal continuous positive airway pressure therapy. *Cardiology* 1991; **79**: 84–92.

24. Suzuki M, Otsuka K, Guilleminault C. Long-term nasal continuous positive airway pressure administration can

normalize hypertension in obstructive sleep apnea patients. *Sleep* 1993; **16**: 545–9.

25. Haentjens P, Van Meerhaeghe A, Moscariello A, et al. The impact of continuous positive airway pressure on blood pressure in patients with obstructive sleep apnea syndrome: evidence from a meta-analysis of placebo-controlled randomized trials. *Arch Intern Med* 2007; **167**: 757–64.

26. Bazzano LA, Khan Z, Reynolds K, et al. Effect of nocturnal nasal continuous positive airway pressure on blood pressure in obstructive sleep apnea. *Hypertension* 2007; **50**: 417–23.

27. Pépin JL, Tamisier R, Barone-Rochette G, et al. Comparison of continuous positive airway pressure and valsartan in hypertensive patients with sleep apnea. *Am J Respir Crit Care Med* 2010; **182**: 954–60.

28. Campos-Rodríguez F, Pérez-Ronchel J, Grilo-Reina A, et al. Long-term effect of continuous positive airway pressure on BP in patients with hypertension and sleep apnea. *Chest* 2007; **132**: 1847–52.

29. Barbé F, Durán-Cantolla J, Capote F, et al. Long-term effect of continuous positive airway pressure in hypertensive patients with sleep apnea. *Am J Respir Crit Care Med* 2010; **181**: 718–26.

30. Faccenda JF, Mackay TW, Boon NA, et al. Randomized placebo-controlled trial of continuous positive airway pressure on blood pressure in the sleep apnea-hypopnea syndrome. *Am J Respir Crit Care Med* 2001; **163**: 344–8.

31. Engleman HM, Gough K, Martin SE, et al. Ambulatory blood pressure on and off continuous positive airway pressure therapy for the sleep apnea/hypopnea syndrome: effects in "non-dippers". *Sleep* 1996; **19**: 378–81.

32. Barbé F, Mayoralas LR, Durán J, et al. Treatment with continuous positive airway pressure is not effective in patients with sleep apnea but no daytime sleepiness: a randomized, controlled trial. *Ann Intern Med* 2001; **134**: 1015–23.

33. Jaimchariyatam N, Rodriguez CL, Budur K. Does CPAP treatment in mild obstructive sleep apnea affect blood pressure? *Sleep Med* 2010; **11**: 837–42.

34. Hui DS, To KW, Ko FW, et al. Nasal CPAP reduces systemic blood pressure in patients with obstructive sleep apnoea and mild sleepiness. *Thorax* 2006; **61**: 1083–90.

35. Brooks D, Horner RL, Kozar LF, et al. Obstructive sleep apnea as a cause of systemic hypertension. Evidence from a canine model. *J Clin Invest* 1997; **99**: 106–9.

36. Wolk R, Shamsuzzaman AS, Somers VK. Obesity, sleep apnea, and hypertension. *Hypertension* 2003; **42**: 1067–74.

37. Narkiewicz K, van de Borne PJ, Cooley RL, et al. Sympathetic activity in obese subjects with and without obstructive sleep apnea. *Circulation* 1998; **98**: 772–6.

38. Phillips BG, Kato M, Narkiewicz K, et al. Increases in leptin levels, sympathetic drive, and weight gain in obstructive sleep apnea. *Am J Physiol* 2000; **279**: H234–7.

39. Di Guardo A, Profeta G, Crisafulli C, et al. Obstructive sleep apnoea in patients with obesity and hypertension. *Br J Gen Pract* 2010; **60**: 325–8.

40. Narkiewicz K, Kato M, Phillips BG, et al. Nocturnal continuous positive airway pressure decreases daytime sympathetic traffic in obstructive sleep apnea. *Circulation* 1999; **100**: 2332–5.

41. Chin K, Shimizu K, Nakamura T, et al. Changes in intra-abdominal visceral fat and serum leptin levels in patients with obstructive sleep apnea syndrome following nasal continuous positive airway pressure therapy. *Circulation* 1999; **100**: 706–12.

42. Worsnop CJ, Naughton MT, Barter CE, et al. The prevalence of obstructive sleep apnea in hypertensives. *Am J Respir Crit Care Med* 1998; **157**: 111–15.

43. Kales A, Bixler EO, Cadieux RJ, et al. Sleep apnoea in a hypertensive population. *Lancet* 1984; **2**: 1005–8.

44. Grote L, Hedner J, Peter JH. Sleep-related breathing disorder is an independent risk factor for uncontrolled hypertension. *J Hypertens* 2000; **18**: 679–85.

45. O'Connor GT, Caffo B, Newman AB, et al. Prospective study of sleep-disordered breathing and hypertension: the Sleep Heart Health Study. *Am J Respir Crit Care Med* 2009; **179**: 1159–64.

46. Sharma SK, Agrawal S, Damodaran D, et al. CPAP for the metabolic syndrome in

patients with obstructive sleep apnea. *N Engl J Med* 2011; **365**: 2277–86.

47. Drager LF, Genta PR, Pedrosa RP, et al. Characteristics and predictors of obstructive sleep apnea in patients with systemic hypertension. *Am J Cardiol* 2010; **105**: 1135–9.

48. Venkateswaran S, Shankar P. The prevalence of syndrome Z (the interaction of obstructive sleep apnoea with the metabolic syndrome) in a teaching hospital in Singapore. *Postgrad Med J* 2007; **83**: 329–31.

49. Wilcox I, McNamara SG, Collins FL, et al. "Syndrome Z": the interaction of sleep apnoea, vascular risk factors and heart disease. *Thorax* 1998; **53**: S25–8.

50. Demede M, Pandey A, Zizi F, et al. Resistant hypertension and obstructive sleep apnea in the primary-care setting. *Int J Hypertens* 2011; **2011**: 340929.

51. Pratt-Ubunama MN, Nishizaka MK, Boedefeld RL, et al. Plasma aldosterone is related to severity of obstructive sleep apnea in subjects with resistant hypertension. *Chest* 2007; **131**: 453–9.

52. Dernaika TA, Kinasewitz GT, Tawk MM. Effects of nocturnal continuous positive airway pressure therapy in patients with resistant hypertension and obstructive sleep apnea. *J Clin Sleep Med* 2009; **5**: 103–7.

53. Aronow WS, Fleg JL, Pepine CJ, et al. ACCF/AHA 2011 Expert Consensus Document on Hypertension in the Elderly: a report of the American College of Cardiology Foundation Task Force on Clinical Expert Consensus Documents. *Circulation* 2011; **123**: 2434–506.

54. Chobanian AV, Bakris GL, Black HR, et al. Seventh report of the Joint National Committee on Prevention, Detection, Evaluation, and Treatment of High Blood Pressure. *Hypertension* 2003; **42**: 1206–52.

55. Silva GE, Vana KD, Goodwin JL, et al. Identification of patients with sleep disordered breathing: comparing the four-variable screening tool, STOP, STOP-Bang, and Epworth Sleepiness Scales. *J Clin Sleep Med* 2011; **7**: 467–72.

56. Netzer NC, Stoohs RA, Netzer CM, et al. Using the Berlin Questionnaire to identify patients at risk for the sleep apnea syndrome. *Ann Intern Med* 1999; **131**: 485–91.

57. Chung F, Yegneswaran B, Liao P, et al. STOP questionnaire: a tool to screen patients for obstructive sleep apnea. *Anesthesiology* 2008; **108**: 812–21.

58. Abrishami A, Khajehdehi A, Chung F. A systematic review of screening questionnaires for obstructive sleep apnea. *Can J Anaesth* 2010; **57**: 423–38.

59. Ramachandran SK, Josephs LA. A meta-analysis of clinical screening tests for obstructive sleep apnea. *Anesthesiology* 2009; **110**: 928–39.

60. Gus M, Gonçalves SC, Martinez D, et al. Risk for obstructive sleep apnea by Berlin Questionnaire, but not daytime sleepiness, is associated with resistant hypertension: a case-control study. *Am J Hypertens* 2008; **21**: 832–5.

61. MacMahon S, Peto R, Cutler J, et al. Blood pressure, stroke, and coronary heart disease. Part 1, Prolonged differences in blood pressure: prospective observational studies corrected for the regression dilution bias. *Lancet* 1990; **335**: 765–74.

62. Gotsopoulos H, Kelly JJ, Cistulli PA. Oral appliance therapy reduces blood pressure in obstructive sleep apnea: a randomized, controlled trial. *Sleep* 2004; **27**: 934–41.

63. Otsuka R, Ribeiro de Almeida F, Lowe AA, et al. The effect of oral appliance therapy on blood pressure in patients with obstructive sleep apnea. *Sleep Breath* 2006; **10**: 29–36.

64. Amin R, Anthony L, Somers V, et al. Growth velocity predicts recurrence of sleep-disordered breathing 1 year after adenotonsillectomy. *Am J Respir Crit Care Med* 2008; **177**: 654–9.

65. Horne RS, Yang JS, Walter LM, et al. Elevated blood pressure during sleep and wake in children with sleep-disordered breathing. *Pediatrics* 2011; **128**: e85–92

66. Ng DK, Wong JC, Chan CH, et al. Ambulatory blood pressure before and after adenotonsillectomy in children with obstructive sleep apnea. *Sleep Med* 2010; **11**: 721–5.

67. Bucca CB, Brussino L, Battisti A, et al. Diuretics in obstructive sleep apnea with diastolic heart failure. *Chest* 2007; **132**: 440–6.

68. Yumino D, Redolfi S, Ruttanaumpawan P, et al. Nocturnal rostral fluid shift: a unifying concept for the pathogenesis of obstructive

and central sleep apnea in men with heart failure. *Circulation* 2010; **121**: 1598–605.

69. Friedman O, Bradley TD, Chan CT, et al. Relationship between overnight rostral fluid shift and obstructive sleep apnea in drug-resistant hypertension. *Hypertension* 2010; **56**: 1077–82.

70. Gonzaga CC, Gaddam KK, Ahmed MI, et al. Severity of obstructive sleep apnea is related to aldosterone status in subjects with resistant hypertension. *J Clin Sleep Med* 2010; **6**: 363–8.

71. Champagne K, Schwartzman K, Opatrny L, et al. Obstructive sleep apnoea and its association with gestational hypertension. *Eur Respir J* 2009; **33**: 559–65.

72. Poyares D, Guilleminault C, Hachul H, et al. Pre-eclampsia and nasal CPAP: part 2. Hypertension during pregnancy, chronic snoring, and early nasal CPAP intervention. *Sleep Med* 2007; **9**: 15–21.

73. Franklin KA, Holmgren PA, Jönsson F, et al. Snoring, pregnancy-induced hypertension, and growth retardation of the fetus. *Chest* 2000; **117**: 137–41.

74. Bourjeily G, Ankner G, Mohsenin V. Sleep-disordered breathing in pregnancy. *Clin Chest Med* 2011; **32**: 175–89.

75. Chen YH, Kang JH, Lin CC, et al. Obstructive sleep apnea and the risk of adverse pregnancy outcomes. *Am J Obstet Gynecol* 2012; **206**: 136.e1–5.

76. Amin R, Somers VK, McConnell K, et al. Activity-adjusted 24-hour ambulatory blood pressure and cardiac remodeling in children with sleep disordered breathing. *Hypertension* 2008; **51**: 84–91.

77. Sajkov D, McEvoy RD. Obstructive sleep apnea and pulmonary hypertension. *Prog Cardiovasc Dis* 2009; **51**: 363–70.

78. Minai OA, Ricaurte B, Kaw R, et al. Frequency and impact of pulmonary hypertension in patients with obstructive sleep apnea syndrome. *Am J Cardiol* 2009; **104**: 1300–6.

79. Alchanatis M, Tourkohoriti G, Kakouros S, et al. Daytime pulmonary hypertension in patients with obstructive sleep apnea: the effect of continuous positive airway pressure on pulmonary hemodynamics. *Respiration* 2001; **68**: 566–72.

80. Mokhlesi B, Tulaimat A, Faibussowitsch I, et al. Obesity hypoventilation syndrome: prevalence and predictors in patients with obstructive sleep apnea. *Sleep Breath* 2007; **11**: 117–24.

81. Mokhlesi B, Kryger MH, Grunstein RR. Assessment and management of patients with obesity hypoventilation syndrome. *Proc Am Thorac Soc* 2008; **5**: 218–25.

82. Mokhlesi B. Obesity hypoventilation syndrome: a state-of-the-art review. *Respir Care* 2010; **55**: 1347–62; discussion 1363–5.

83. Colish J, Walker JR, Elmayergi N, et al. Obstructive sleep apnea: effects of continuous positive airway pressure on cardiac remodeling as assessed by cardiac biomarkers, echocardiography, and cardiac MRI. *Chest* 2012; **141**: 674–81.

84. Yilmaz MD, Onrat E, Altuntaş A, et al. The effects of tonsillectomy and adenoidectomy on pulmonary arterial pressure in children. *Am J Otolaryngol* 2005; **26**: 18–21.

85. Duman D, Naiboglu B, Esen HS, et al. Impaired right ventricular function in adenotonsillar hypertrophy. *Int J Cardiovasc Imaging* 2008; **24**: 261–7.

Sleep apnea, stroke risk factors, and the arousal response

Mark Eric Dyken, George B. Richerson and
Kyoung Bin Im

Introduction

Evidence suggests that untreated obstructive sleep apnea (OSA) is a significant health risk for the development of hypertension, cardiovascular disease, and stroke. Sleep-related abnormal obstructive respiratory events can lead to significant hypoxemia, hypercapnia, and simultaneous elevations in sympathetic and parasympathetic activity, with significant variations in blood pressure, tachycardia/bradycardia, and asystole. Termination of untreated OSA-related events is generally dependent upon the arousal response. Some experts have hypothesized that dysfunction of the arousal response in OSA may, in some cases, allow for a cause-and-effect relationship between untreated OSA and stroke, cardiac dysrhythmia, and death.

Untreated obstructive sleep apnea as a risk factor for stroke

Transient ischemic attack reports

A transient ischemic attack (TIA; "ministroke") is a focal neurological deficit that resolves within 24 hours [1]. As an estimated 15% of strokes are preceded by TIA, with a 90-day risk of up to 17.3%, some experts have used polysomnography (PSG) investigations of subjects with TIA as indirect evidence to support a cause-and-effect relationship between OSA and stroke [1–3]. One such case consisted of associated transient episodes of left hemiplegia, ophthalmoplegia, and Babinski signs upon awakening [4]. The PSG showed each event was preceded by an obstructive apnea.

Another case report involved an obese, sleepy, 64-year-old woman with a history of loud snoring who awoke on one occasion with a motor aphasia, mild dizziness, and lethargy that resolved over a three-hour period [5]. The PSG analysis revealed an apnea/hypopnea index (AHI) of 83.4 events/hour, with oxygen desaturations of <50% that were frequently associated with a clear tachycardia/bradycardia with heart rate changes from 30 to 50 beats per minute. The use of continuous positive airway pressure (CPAP) therapy was followed by a resolution of any further TIAs.

In a 1996 study of 13 consecutively encountered subjects with TIA, OSA was diagnosed in 69% of subjects with TIA and in only 16% of controls [6]. Another study of 86 subjects with TIA revealed no significant difference between the mean (+/−SD) AHIs of the TIA (21+/−17.0) and control (21+/−14.4 events/h) groups [7].

Although OSA is not considered a proven risk factor for TIA, these anecdotal reports have suggested to some that OSA might predispose to TIA [6,7]. In such cases, CPAP might be considered as stroke prophylaxis [4,5].

Cohort studies

Large population- and clinic-based cohort studies have addressed the incidence of stroke in a variety of subject groups suffering from OSA (Table 5.1).

Population-based studies

In 2005, a report was published that addressed a 12-year period during which data was gathered from a stratified random sample [8]. A cross-sectional analysis, utilizing logistic regression, involving 1475 adult subjects between 30 and 60 years of age showed that a baseline AHI of >20 events/h independently increased the odds ratio (OR) for stroke (3.83; 95% CI, 1.17–12.56; P=0.03) compared to the reference group with an AHI of <5 events/h, after adjusting for confounding factors (age, gender, body mass index [BMI], alcohol, smoking, diabetes mellitus, and hypertension).

From the original population, a longitudinal analysis of 1189 individuals tested whether sleep-disordered breathing (SDB) was associated with increased incident stroke at four-year intervals (4, 8, and 12 years). In a model controlled for age and gender, subjects with a baseline AHI of >20 events/h had a significantly higher OR for incident stroke compared to the reference group (4.48; 95% CI, 1.31–15.33; P=0.02).

A 2001 study examined the cross-sectional association between SDB and self-reported cardiovascular disease (CVD) in 6424 subjects with unattended home PSGs [9]. Mild to moderate SDB was highly prevalent with a median AHI of 4.4 events/h, with an inter-quartile range of 1.3–11.0. Sixteen percent (n=1023) of the subjects reported one or more manifestation(s) of CVD defined as myocardial infarction, angina, coronary revascular-ization procedure, heart failure, or stroke. The relative odds value (95% CI) of prevalent stroke (upper versus lower AHI quartile) was 1.58 (1.02–22.46). It was emphasized that these findings suggested SDB had modest to moderate effects on heterogeneous manifest-ations of CVD within a range of AHI values generally considered as normal or only mildly elevated.

Clinic-based studies

In 2005, an observational cohort study utilized 1022 subjects with suspected SDB, and compared the combined risk of developing composite stroke, TIA, or death from any cause in a group of 697 individuals with OSA (AHI >5 events/h), to subjects with an AHI of <5 events/h [10]. Many apneics were treated during the study (diet, positive airway pressure therapy, or upper-airway surgery).

Over a 3.3- to 3.4-year follow-up period, data from 842 subjects revealed 22 incident strokes and/or TIAs and 50 deaths in the OSA group, with only 2 total incident strokes and/or TIAs and 14 deaths in the comparison group. Even after adjusting for age, gender, race, smoking, BMI, diabetes, hyperlipidemia, atrial fibrillation, and hypertension, OSA was still found to be associated with a significant risk for composite stroke, TIA, or death (hazard ratio, 1.97; 95% CI, 1.12–3.48; P=0.01). A trend analysis determined that an increase in the severity of OSA was associated with an increased risk of stroke, TIA, or death from any cause (P=0.005).

Table 5.1. Obstructive sleep apnea and stroke risk: incidence studies

Incidence studies Authors/year	Subjects studied	Population size	AHI used to define SDB group	SDB prevalence	AHI used to define comparison group	Mean follow-up period (years)	Group outcome: total number of subjects in a given group with outcome	Risk estimate of SDB as risk factor for outcome (95% CI)
Arzt et al., 2005 [8]	–Population based –General adult30 to 60 years	†1475 ††1189	≥20	7% (n = 99)	<5	3 intervals of 4 years	Stroke SDB = 4 Comparison = 9	*OR=4.48 (1.31–15.33; P=0.02)
Yaggi et al., 2005 [10]	–Clinic based –Referred for suspected SDB: ≥50 years	1022	≥5	68% (n = 697)	<5	3.4; SDB 3.3; CG	Stroke, TIA, or death SDB = 72 Comparison = 16	**HR=1.97 (1.12–3.48; P=0.01)
Muñoz et al., 2006 [11]	–Clinic based –Random sample, noninstitutional: elderly, 70 to 100 years	394	≥30	25% (n = 98)	< 0	4.5	TIA or ischemic stroke SDB = 9 Comparison = 11	***HR=2.52 (1.04–6.1; P=0.04)
Valham et al., 2008 [12]	–Clinic based –Symptomatic angina and CAD	392	≥5	54% (n = 211)	<5	10.0	Stroke SDB = 38 Comparison = 9	****HR=2.89 (1.37–6.09; P=0.005)
Redline et al., 2010 [13]	–Community based: ≥40 years	5422	>15	Male 44% (n = 1095) Female 24% (n = 720)	<4.1	8.7	Ischemic stroke Male SDB = 54 Female SDB = 37	Male: ***** HR=2.86 (1.1–7.4) Female: ****** A 2% increase in HR (0–5) after threshold OAHI of 25

AHI, apnea/hypopnea index = the average number of apneas and hypopneas per hour of sleep; SDB, sleep-disordered breathing; CI, confidence interval; CAD, coronary artery disease; CG, comparison group; TIA, transient ischemic attack; P, probability; OR, odds ratio; HR, hazard ratio; OAHI, obstructive apnea/hypopnea index;

† original population providing original cross-sectional prevalence data;

†† population used for longitudinal analysis of incident stroke;

* in a model adjusted for age and gender;

** in a model adjusted for age, gender, race, smoking, BMI, diabetes mellitus, hyperlipidemia, atrial fibrillation, and hypertension;

*** in a model adjusted for gender;

**** in a model adjusted for age, BMI, left ventricular function, diabetes, gender, intervention, hypertension, atrial fibrillation, previous stroke or TIA.

***** in a model for male subjects comparing the risk for ischemic stroke and the OAHI in the top quartile (quartile IV; OAHI >19) to the lowest quartile (quartile I; OAHI <4.1 events/h) of the overall population studied;

****** in a model using non-linear, covariate adjusted associations between OAHI and the female gender. (Modified from Table 1 in Dyken MD, Im KB. Obstructive sleep apnea and stroke. Chest 2009; **136**: 1668–77, with permission).

In 2006, a study was performed on a noninstitutionalized population of elderly subjects (age range, 70–100 yr; median, 77.28 yr), drawn from a random one-stage cluster sampling stratified by census areas, age, and gender [11]. A baseline AHI of >30 events/h, after adjusting for gender, was found to be a risk factor for incident TIA or ischemic stroke with a hazard ratio of 2.52 (95% CI, 1.04–6.1; P=0.04).

In 2008, a study was performed on a population of people 70 years of age and younger, with symptomatic angina pectoris and coronary artery disease (verified by coronary angiography and left ventriculography) [12]. Three hundred and ninety-two patients were randomly selected for modified PSG assessments (without electroencephalography [EEG]), using a pressure-sensitive bed to detect respiratory movements.

On the first evaluation, 54% of the subjects were found to have sleep apnea defined as an AHI of >5 events/h. All subjects were followed over 10 years (nine received treatment for OSA); stroke developed in 47 (12%). The initial presence of sleep apnea was associated with an increased risk of stroke with a hazard ratio of 2.89 (95% CI, 1.37–6.09; P=005) that was independent of age, gender, BMI, smoking, left ventricular function, diabetes mellitus, hypertension, atrial fibrillation, previous stroke or TIA, or treatment intervention for OSA. Subjects with an AHI of >5 and <15, and those with an AHI of >15 events/h, respectively, had 2.44- (59% CI, 1.08–5.52; P=0.011) and 3.56- (95% CI, 1.56–8.16; P=0.011) times increased risk of stroke compared to those without apnea, independent of confounders.

Finally, in 2010 the results from the Sleep Heart Health Study were published [13]. Five thousand four hundred and twenty-two participants, without a history of stroke, were followed for a median of 8.7 years, after which 193 new ischemic strokes were observed. There was a significant positive association between ischemic strokes and the obstructive apnea/hypopnea index (OAHI). In men with an OAHI of >19.1 events/h (the top quartile), there was a greater risk for stroke with an adjusted hazard ratio of 2.86 (95% CI, 1.1–7.4) when compared to men with an OAHI of <4.1 events/h (quartile I). In women, following adjustment for covariates that included BMI, race, smoking, systolic blood pressure, antihypertensive medication, and diabetes mellitus, stroke risk was not associated with the OAHI quartile or oxygen desaturation levels. Nevertheless, the authors explored non-linear, covariate-adjusted associations with the OSA exposures and interactions with gender and found that in women there was a 2% increase (95% CI, 0–5) in stroke hazard ratio with each unit increment in OAHI after a threshold of 25 events/h.

Cohort studies to date have looked at a variety of populations using variable PSG methodologies, OSA definitions, and statistical analyses, and have frequently addressed stroke risk in combination with other pathologies. Nevertheless, the data suggests that, in the general adult population, untreated OSA with a severity approximated by an AHI of >20 events/h is a risk factor for stroke [8,13].

Treatment versus non-treatment

In 1996, we attempted to perform a four-year reassessment of all 24 patients we had originally studied in 1992 with PSG after recent stroke and each gender- and age-matched control subject that was associated with that research [14,15]. Reassessments were made on all individuals with stroke and on all but three of the controls (subjects had moved, leaving no contact information). The only patients with stroke who were subsequently found to have died (n=5) also suffered from OSA. Of these individuals, only one used CPAP, and that patient died from urosepsis. The only control subject who died was a male without significant OSA whose cause of death was related to prostatic carcinoma. A retrospective analysis of the PSG data showed mean AHIs of 22.1 and 41.3 events/h for stroke patients found to be alive and dead at follow-up, respectively. These findings suggested that the diagnosis and severity of OSA in stroke might be associated with a greater risk of mortality.

Cause-and-effect can be proven utilizing prospective, treatment versus non-treatment studies. In 1990, the results of a seven-year study were published where 198 patients with OSA were treated with tracheostomy (71 subjects) or weight loss only (127 individuals) [16,17]. At follow-up, 1.2% of the tracheostomy group had suffered a stroke (2.8% died), whereas 5.2% of the weight-loss group had experienced a new stroke (17.3% died, 11% from vascular causes). These results suggest that under-treated OSA leads to higher morbidity and mortality from stroke.

Potential mechanisms for obstructive sleep apnea-induced stroke

The metabolic syndrome

Obstructive sleep apnea, obesity, hypertension, and insulin resistance/diabetes mellitus are independently associated with multiple risk factors for stroke that are summarized in the metabolic syndrome [1,18,19]. A strong association has been shown between the metabolic syndrome and OSA [20–25]. Up to 53% of newly diagnosed apneics have the metabolic syndrome [20]. One cross-sectional case-control study found that the metabolic syndrome is significantly more common in OSA than in controls (49.5% versus 22.0% for men, P<0.01; 32.0% versus 6.7% for women, P<0.01) [21]. Obstructive sleep apnea increases the odds of having the metabolic syndrome from five- to nine-fold [22,23].

Obstructive sleep apnea is independently associated with obesity, hypertension, and insulin resistance/diabetes mellitus; three stroke risk factors of the metabolic syndrome [1,18,19,26]. An increase in BMI by one standard deviation increases the OR for SDB (as defined by an AHI $\geq$5 events/h) by 4.17 [27]. One prospective, population-based study over four years showed that the OR of a subject with an AHI between 5.0 and 14.9 versus $\geq$15.0 events/h for developing hypertension was two- versus three-times greater, respectively, than for someone without the diagnosis of apnea [28]. A recent community-based, cross-sectional study of 69 non-diabetic subjects revealed that those with mild and moderately severe OSA (not specifically defined) had significantly reduced insulin sensitivities (38.5% and 51.2%, respectively) compared to normal subjects without apnea (those with an AHI of <5 events/h), independent of age, gender, race, and percentage of total and visceral body fat [29].

Autonomic activity

The hypothesis that OSA-induced hypertension can lead to stroke is supported by micro-neurographic studies that directly measured efferent sympathetic neural activity (SNA) [30,31]. Obstructive sleep apnea can elevate SNA as a result of the reflex effects of hypoxia, hypercapnia, and decreased input from thoracic stretch receptors (Figures 5.1 and 5.2) [32]. In 10 subjects with OSA, SNA increased by 246% during the last 10 seconds of apneic events, in association with a mean blood pressure increase from 92 mmHg in the waking state to 127 mmHg in REM sleep [33]. Persistently elevated waking sympathetic tone suggests OSA can induce chronic changes that might also predispose to stroke [31,33].

A mixed apnea

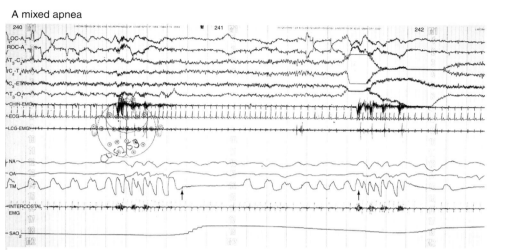

Figure 5.1. A polysomnography tracing (paper speed 10 mm/sec) has been reduced to correspond to a temporally related microneurographic tracing (see Figure 5.3; paper speed 5 mm/sec). Arrows indicate a prolonged mixed apnea of approximately 26-second duration occurring during rapid eye movement (REM) sleep, associated with severe oxygen desaturation. LOC, left outer canthus; ROC, right outer canthus; T, temporal; C, central; ET, ears tied; O, occipital; EMG, electromyogram; NA, nasal airflow; OA, oral airflow; TM, thoracic movement; SAO$_2$, oxygen saturation. (Modified from Figure 2 in Dyken [31], with permission.)

A microneurographic study during a mixed apnea

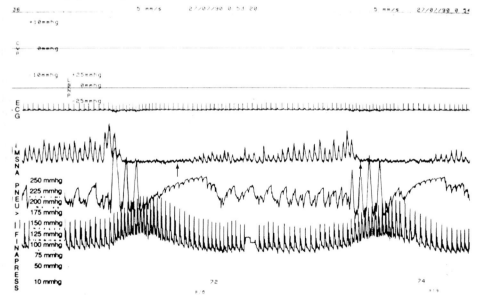

Figure 5.2. The arrows in this microneurographic tracing recorded from the peroneal nerve indicate a gradual elevation of efferent nerve activity during a mixed apnea. The activity peak is immediately followed by cessation of the apnea, with a subsequent marked elevation of arterial blood pressure to 215/130 mmHg from a baseline of 135/80 mmHg. MSNA, muscle sympathetic nerve activity; Pneu, chest excursion; Finapress, fingertip blood pressure. (Modified from Figure 3 in Dyken [31], with permission.)

Autonomic effects could contribute to the high prevalence of cardiac arrhythmias reported in up to 48% of apneics [34–36]. Obstructive apneas can lead to excessive parasympathetic responses associated with inspiring against a closed glottis and hypoxemia, with recurrent prolonged episodes of sinus arrest and dramatic reductions in blood pressure that have been documented to decrease from 180/100 mmHg (prior to obstructions) to systolic pressures of <50 mmHg during obstructions [37].

Patients with atrial fibrillation are at 49% risk for having OSA and CPAP noncompliance is associated with a greater recurrence rate of atrial fibrillation after cardioversion [38,39]. Atrial fibrillation, a strong risk factor for stroke, might contribute to stroke in some patients with OSA [1].

Circadian rhythms

Our group hypothesized that if stroke has an equal probability of occurring at any time during a 24-hour period, 33% should occur during the stereotypical eight-hour episode of nocturnal sleep [15]. However, stroke tends to occur in the early morning hours [40]. In our prospective prevalence study of stroke, a higher than expected percentage of apneics suffered strokes during sleep (54%; P=0.0304) [15].

Rapid eye movement sleep

The most prolonged period of rapid eye movement (REM or stage R) sleep (the early morning) coincides with the greatest circadian risk for stroke. The muscular paresis that is normally associated with REM sleep generally worsens OSA and may potentiate the risk for stroke during this period. Rapid eye movement sleep is also normally associated with a relative elevation of SNA and blood pressures that tend to reach waking levels, and intermittently demonstrate pressure surges in association with phasic REM-related muscle twitches [41,42]. Amplification of these negative autonomic phenomena has been documented in OSA.

Cerebral blood flow normally increases in REM sleep, whereas obstructive apneic events increase intracranial pressure and reduce cerebral perfusion pressure [43,44]. In patients with severe OSA, these elements, when combined with REM-related SNA elevation and concomitant blood pressure instability, might provide for a synergism that could predispose to stroke.

Early morning is normally associated with low fibrinolytic activity and high levels of catecholamines, blood viscosity, and platelet activity and aggregability; a time when REM-related SNA activation and hemodynamic instability might potentiate platelet aggregation and plaque development [45]. In the hematological milieu, elevation of catecholamines and platelet activation in association with OSA may further increase thrombus and embolus formation, and the subsequent risk for stroke [46,47].

Increased levels of two platelet activation proteins, soluble CD40 ligand (sCD40L) and soluble P-selectin (sP-selectin), have been linked to silent brain infarctions (SBI) [48]. A study utilized brain MRIs to show SBI in 25% of subjects with moderate to severe OSA and in only 6.7% of controls [48]. Serum levels of sCD40L and sP-selectin were significantly higher in apneics compared to controls, and treatment with CPAP led to a significant reduction of these platelet activation proteins.

The arousal phenomena

Arousal from non-rapid eye movement (NREM or N) stages N1, N2, and N3 sleep, as defined in the American Academy of Sleep Medicine (AASM) manual for the scoring of sleep and associated events [49], uses a three-second rule where there is an abrupt shift of EEG frequency that includes alpha, theta, and/or frequencies of >16 Hz (but not sleep spindles) lasting at least three seconds, with at least 10 seconds of stable sleep preceding the change. Arousal from REM sleep also requires a concurrent increase in submental electromyographic activity of at least one second's duration [49]. However, this definition is consensus-based and may underestimate the impact of disruptive influences on sleep [50].

Studies in normal subjects and sleep apneic patients suggest that upper airway occlusion induces arousal from NREM sleep once the level of inspiratory effort reaches a certain value (the arousal threshold), which varies among individuals [51]. In one case study, an impaired arousal response during the sleep of a patient with OSA was suspected to prolong apneas, leading to a flattening of the EEG and generalized tonic spasms, which were described as "cerebral anoxic attacks" [52]. Our group subsequently hypothesized that an increase in the arousal threshold may predispose critically ill patients with OSA to prolonged apneas and death during sleep. We reported on two cases where PSG-documented OSA resulted in EEG changes compatible with cerebral hypoxemia, with subsequent transient encephalopathy in one instance and death in the other (Figures 5.3, 5.4, and 5.5) [53].

The arousal threshold to hypoxia and hypercapnia can be increased by short-term sleep deprivation [54]. In one study it was stated that as sleep deprivation is common in acutely ill patients, they could only "speculate at this time as to the clinical significance of these findings as they apply to the patient with a precarious respiratory status." [54]. Investigators have shown that OSA, in and of itself, increases the arousal threshold [51]. They hypothesized that this is the result of sleep fragmentation and possibly due to other factors such as hypoxemia [51].

In addition, an immediate effect of the initial use of CPAP therapy is to further increase the arousal threshold [55]. Twelve patients with OSA were studied on consecutive nights, without and with CPAP [55]. Treatment resulted in an up to a 370% mean increase in the percentage of time spent in stage 3 NREM (N3) sleep, longer REM sleep periods and rapid-eye-movement bursts, and an increase in REM sleep phasic muscle twitching. It has been hypothesized that this "rebound" sleep is responsible for a "marked depression of the patient's arousability" and leaves them "vulnerable to potential life-threatening hypoxemia." [56]. Experts have stated that "This phenomenon can occur in patients usually with severe sleep apnea and carbon dioxide retention when a subcritical level of CPAP is selected, resulting in partial upper airway obstruction during these abnormally long episodes of REM sleep." [53,56].

Mechanisms of arousal during obstructive sleep apnea

Each episode of sleep apnea typically terminates with an arousal. Patients are usually not aware that they wake up, but this transient arousal is an important protective reflex that leads to unconscious relief of the upper airway obstruction as well as an increase in tidal volume and respiratory frequency. Without this arousal, it is likely that the apnea would not terminate. Thus, there is great interest in the mechanisms of the arousal that occurs in response to apnea in patients with OSA.

A hypoxemic
encephalopathic EEG
pattern following a
prolonged obstructive
apnea

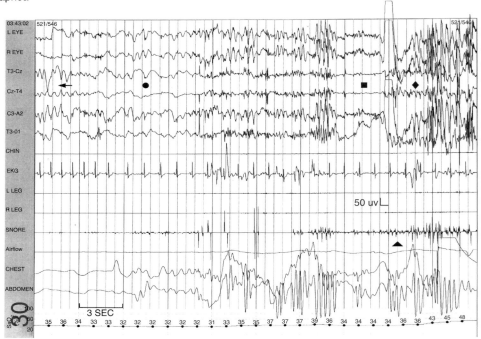

Figure 5.3. This patient suffered a prolonged obstructive apnea that eventually resulted in a sudden electroencephalogram (EEG) change from a classic rapid eye movement (REM) sawtooth pattern (arrow) to a poorly organized, diffuse delta slow-wave pattern (closed circle), followed by a general flattening of all activity (square) that led to attempts to arouse the patient (as evidenced by the diffuse movement artifact [diamond]). Nevertheless, persistent obstruction (triangle) necessitated emergency rescue breathing maneuvers. Persistent EEG flattening followed by slowing and eventual recovery of normal waking patterns was appreciated in subsequent epochs. L, left; R, right; T, temporal; C, central; O, occipital; CHIN, mentalis EMG; L Leg, left anterior tibialis EMG; R LEG, right anterior tibialis EMG; SNORE, snoring microphone; ABDOMEN, abdominal effort; SaO$_2$ (%), oxygen saturation. (Modified from Figure 1 in Dyken et al. [53], with permission.)

During apnea there are several stimuli that are well known to be able to induce arousal, including hypercapnia, hypoxia, and increased airway resistance.

Hypercapnia

An increase in partial pressure of carbon dioxide (PaCO$_2$) in arterial blood is a powerful stimulus for arousal. When a healthy human subject is exposed to 8% CO$_2$ in the ambient air while they are sleeping, they typically wake up within 60 seconds [57]. Similar effects are seen in other mammals. For example, sleeping mice have a dose-dependent decrease in arousal latency in response to an increase in ambient CO$_2$ from 0% (normal) to between 3% and 10% [58]. Arousal occurs in less than 60 seconds in response to 7% CO$_2$.

A hypoxemic encephalopathic EEG pattern following a prolonged obstructive apnea

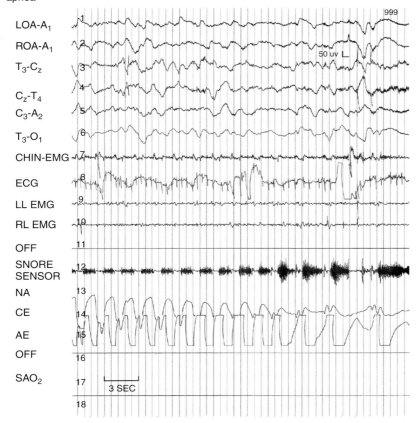

Figure 5.4. An 80-year-old man with multiple medical problems, who was admitted with exacerbation of pulmonary and cardiac disease under a do-not-resuscitate/do-not-intubate status (for whom signed consent had been given for polysomnography as part of an IRB-approved study), had a 30-second obstruction that was associated with a low SaO_2 of 12%. At that time the EEG showed progressive development of a disorganized slow-wave pattern over a 2½-minute period, followed by ECS [electrocerebral silence] (using a recording sensitivity of 1.0 μV/mm). A_1 left ear reference; A_2, right ear reference; T, temporal; C, central; O, occipital; LL, left leg; RL, right leg; NA, nasal airflow; CE, chest effort; AE, abdominal effort; SAO_2, oxygen saturation. (Modified from Figures 19–10 in Dyken ME, Afifi AK, Im KB. Stroke in sleep. In Chokroverty S, Sahota P, eds. *Acute and Emergent Events in Sleep Disorders*. New York, NY: Oxford University Press, 2011, 328–48, with permission.)

Arousal to CO_2 is mediated by serotonin neurons. These neurons, located within the raphe nuclei of the brainstem, are closely associated with large branches of the basilar artery [59]. They are sensors of arterial CO_2, responding indirectly to changes in brain pH by increasing their excitatory drive to other neurons that mediate arousal, possibly including those in the thalamus and cortex [60]. Transgenic mice in which all serotonin neurons are deleted from the brain can sometimes survive to adulthood. Those that survive

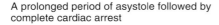

A prolonged period of asystole followed by
complete cardiac arrest

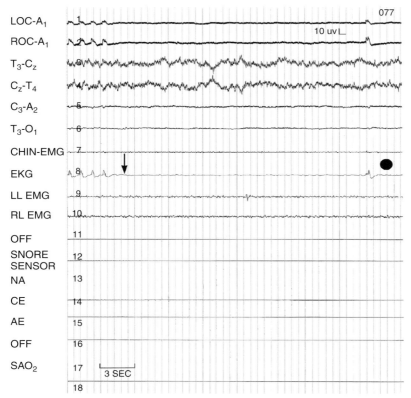

Figure 5.5. After the patient in Figure 5.4 (upon whom no resuscitative therapeutic interventions were allowed) had a final series of apneic events, no discernible electroencephalographic (EEG) activity was captured while utilizing a recording sensitivity or 1.0 μV/mm. A prolonged period of asystole (arrow) was followed by cardiac arrest, at which time the patient was declared dead (closed circle). LOC, left outer canthus; A$_1$, left ear reference; A$_2$, right ear reference; T, temporal; C, central; O, occipital; LL, left leg; RL, right leg; NA, nasal airflow; CE, chest effort; AE, abdominal effort; SA0$_2$, oxygen saturation. (Modified from Figure 2 in Dyken et al. [53], with permission.)

do not wake up from sleep in response to an increase in CO_2 to as high as 10% [58]. However, they wake normally in response to sound, air puffs, or a decrease in O_2. Their baseline sleep is disrupted, as previously reported, with chemical depletion of serotonin [61]. However, this is not because of a direct effect on sleep, but is indirectly due to a decrease in body temperature when animals were studied at an ambient temperature of 23°C. These serotonin-neuron deficient animals have a coexisting defect in thermoregulation, and their baseline sleep is normal as long as they are kept at a thermoneutral ambient temperature of 33°C.

It is not known whether there are individual differences in serotonin neuron function in humans that lead to defects in arousal to hypercapnia. It is also not known whether arousal to CO_2 is affected by drugs that affect the serotonin system, such as selective serotonin reuptake inhibitors (SSRIs). However, SSRIs and ondansetron have both been shown to reduce the

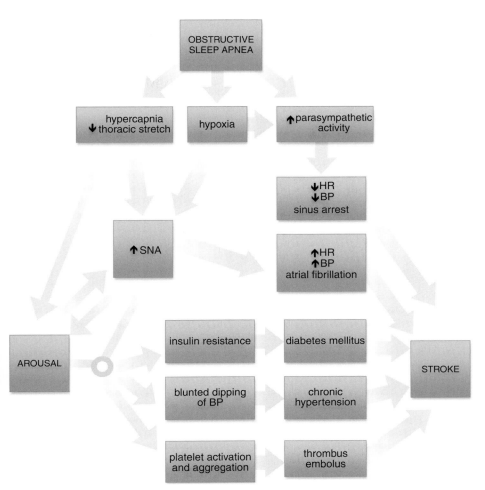

Figure 5.6. This simplified diagram highlights some of the major suspected factors linking obstructive sleep apnea, arousal, and stroke. Obstructive sleep apnea can lead to autonomic instability. Inspiration against a closed airway with hypoxemia can increase parasympathetic activity, potentially leading to bradycardia, sinus arrest, and hypotensive events. Increased sympathetic neural activity (SNA) from the reflex effects of hypoxia, hypercapnia, and decreased input from thoracic stretch receptors can lead to tachycardia, blood pressure (BP) surges, and potentially arrhythmias such as atrial fibrillation. While an acute arousal can be protective in preventing untoward effects of a single prolonged apnea, chronic concomitant SNA elevations have been hypothesized to help explain the known associations with a variety of stroke risk factors, including the development of thrombus/emboli, diabetes mellitus, and chronic hypertension. HR, heart rate.

AHI of patients with OSA [62], and OSA has been found to be more prevalent in individuals who have been users of methylenedioxymethamphetamine (MDMA; "Ecstasy"), a recreational drug that causes chronic impairment of serotonin neuron function [63]. These results could be due to effects on respiratory control mechanisms, but it is also possible that arousal in patients with OSA is influenced by medications that influence serotonin system function. Likewise, there may be differences in hypercapnic arousal due to genetic variations that influence the serotonin system.

Hypoxia and the workload of breathing

Arousal during apnea is also induced by a variety of other factors. For example, inhalation of hypoxic air can induce arousal in the absence of hypercapnia [64]. The reduction in PaO_2 is sensed by the peripheral arterial chemoreceptors in the carotid and aortic bodies, but the central mechanisms are less clearly understood. They do not rely on serotonergic neurons [58], but they may involve other neurons of the raphe nuclei [65] as well as the nucleus tractus solitarius and other brainstem nuclei.

Arousal can also be induced by an increase in the work of breathing that occurs in response to airway occlusion [66]. This is an inevitable consequence of upper airway obstruction in OSA. Curiously, arousal does not occur at the onset of an apnea, even though airway obstruction occurs early. This implies that the hypoxia and hypercapnia that develop over time must be critical factors in the arousal phenomenon.

Conclusion

Cohort studies have shown OSA to be a risk factor for stroke. Obstructive sleep apnea is associated with a variety of stroke risk factors that may independently contribute to stroke risk (Figure 5.6). This suggests the potential for a cause-and-effect relationship between untreated OSA and stroke in some cases. There are anecdotal reports that indicate that depression of the arousal phenomena, in some select patient populations with OSA, might provide for a predisposition to stroke and death due to the effects of sustained hypoxemia and hypercapnia.

References

1. Lloyd-Jones D, Adams R, Mercedes C, et al. Heart disease and stroke statistics-2009 update. A report from the American Heart Association Statistics Committee and Stroke Statistics Subcommittee. *Circulation* 2009; **119**: e21–181.

2. Ovbiagele B, Kidwell CS, Saver JL. Epidemiological impact in the United States of a tissue-based definition of transient ischemic attack. *Stroke* 2003; **34**: 919–24.

3. Kleinddorfer D, Panagos P, Pancioli A, et al. Incidence and short-term prognosis of transient ischemic attack in a population based study. *Stroke* 2005; **36**: 720–3.

4. Rivest J, Reiher J. Transient ischemic attacks triggered by symptomatic sleep apneas [abstract]. *Stroke* 1987; **18**: 293.

5. Pressman MR, Schetman WR, Figueroa WG, et al. Transient ischemic attacks and minor stroke during sleep. *Stroke* 1995; **26**: 2361–5.

6. Bassetti C, Aldrich MS, Chervin RD, et al. Sleep apnea in patients with transient ischemic attack and stroke: a prospective study of 59 patients. *Neurology* 1996; **47**: 1167–73.

7. McArdle N, Riha RL, Vennelle M, et al. Sleep-disordered breathing as a risk factor for cerebrovascular disease; a case-control study in patients with transient ischemic attacks. *Stroke* 2003; **34**: 2916–21.

8. Arzt M, Young T, Finn L, et al. Association of sleep-disordered breathing and the occurrence of stroke. *Am J Resp Crit Care Med* 2005; **172**: 1147–51.

9. Shahar E, Whitney CW, Redline S, et al. Sleep-disordered breathing and cardiovascular disease. Cross-sectional results of the Sleep Heart Health Study. *Am J Resp Crit Care Med* 2001; **163**: 19–25.

10. Yaggi KH, Concato J, Kernan WN, et al. Obstructive sleep apnea as a risk factor for stroke and death. *N Engl J Med* 2005; **19**: 2034–41.

11. Muñoz R, Durán-Cantolla J, Martínez-Vila E, et al. Severe sleep apnea and risk of ischemic stroke in the elderly. *Stroke* 2006; **37**: 2317–21.

12. Valham F, Mooe T, Rabben T, et al. Increased risk of stroke in patients with coronary artery disease and sleep apnea: a

10-year follow-up. *Circulation* 2008; **118**: 955–60.

13. Redline S, Yenokyan G, Gottlieb DJ, et al. Obstructive sleep apnea-hypopnea and incident stroke; The Sleep Heart Health Study. *Am J Respir Crit Care Med* 2010; **182**: 269–77.

14. Dyken ME, Somers VK, Yamada T, et al. Investigating the relationship between sleep apnea and stroke [abstract]. *Sleep Res* 1992; **21**: 30.

15. Dyken ME, Somers VK, Yamada T, et al. Investigating the relationship between stroke and obstructive sleep apnea. *Stroke* 1996; **27**: 401–7.

16. Partinen M, Jamieson A, Guilleminault C. Long-term outcome for obstructive sleep apnea syndrome patients: mortality. *Chest* 1988; **94**: 1200–4.

17. Partinen M, Guilleminault C. Daytime sleepiness and vascular morbidity at seven-year follow-up in obstructive sleep apnea patients. *Chest* 1990; **97**: 27–32.

18. Roger VL, Go AS, Lloyd-Jones D, et al. Heart disease and stroke statistics – 2012 update: a report from the American Heart Association (available online; http://circ. ahajournals.org/content/early/2011/12/15/ CIR.0b013e31823ac046).

19. Rundek T, Gardener H, Xu Q, et al. Insulin resistance and risk of ischemic stroke among nondiabetic individuals from the Northern Manhattan Study. *Arch Neurol* 2010; **67**: 1195–200.

20. Ambrosetti M, Lucioni AM, Conti S, et al. Metabolic syndrome in obstructive sleep apnea and related cardiovascular risk. *J Cardiovasc Med* 2006; **7**: 826–9.

21. Sasanabe R, Banno K, Otake K, et al. Metabolic syndrome in Japanese patients with obstructive sleep apnea syndrome. *Hypertens Res* 2006; **29**: 315–22.

22. Lam JC, Lam B, Lam CL, et al. Obstructive sleep apnea and the metabolic syndrome in community-based Chinese adults in Hong Kong. *Respir Med* 2006; **100**: 980–7.

23. Coughlin SR, Mawdsley L, Mugarza JA, et al. Obstructive sleep apnoea is independently associated with an increased prevalence of metabolic syndrome. *Eur Heart J* 2004; **25**: 735–41.

24. Kono M, Tatsumi K, Saibara T, et al. Obstructive sleep apnea syndrome is associated with some components of metabolic syndrome. *Chest* 2007; **131**: 1387–92.

25. Vgontzas AN, Bixler EO, Chrousos GP. Sleep apnea is a manifestation of the metabolic syndrome. *Sleep Med Rev* 2005; **9**: 211–24.

26. Tishler PV, Larkin EK, Schluchter MD, et al. Incidence of sleep-disordered breathing in an urban adult population. *JAMA* 2003; **289**: 2230–7.

27. Young T, Palta M, Dempsey J, et al. The occurrence of sleep disordered breathing among middle-aged adults. *N Engl J Med* 1993; **328**: 1230–5.

28. Peppard PE, Young T, Palta M, et al. Prospective study of the association between sleep-disordered breathing and hypertension. *N Engl J Med* 2000; **342**: 1378–84.

29. Aurora RN, Polak J, Punjabi NM, et al. Obstructive sleep apnea is associated with insulin resistance independent of visceral fat. *Am J Respir Crit Care Med* 2011; **183**: A6075.

30. Dyken ME, Somers VK, Yamada T. Hemorrhagic stroke; part of the natural history of severe obstructive sleep apnea [abstract]? *Sleep Res* 1991; **20**: 371.

31. Dyken ME. Cerebrovascular disease and sleep apnea. In: Bradley DT, Floras JS, eds. *Sleep Disorders and Cardiovascular and Cerebrovascular Disease*. New York, NY: Marcel Dekker, 2000, 285–306.

32. Somers VK, Mark AL, Abboud FM. Sympathetic activation by hypoxia and hypercapnia. Implications for sleep apnea [abstract]. *Clin Exp Hypertens* 1988; A**10**: 413–22.

33. Somers VK, Dyken ME, Clary MP, et al. Sympathetic neural mechanisms in obstructive sleep apnea. *J Clin Invest* 1995; **96**: 1897–904.

34. Somers VK, Dyken ME, Skinner JL. Autonomic and hemodynamic responses and interactions during the Mueller maneuver in humans. *J Auton Nerv Syst* 1993; **44**: 253–9.

35. Wolk R, Somers VK. Obesity-related cardiovascular disease: implications of

obstructive sleep apnea. *Diabetes Obes Metab* 2006; **8**: 250–60.

36. Guilleminault C, Connolly SJ, Winkle RA. Cardiac arrhythmia and conduction disturbances during sleep in 400 patients with sleep apnea syndrome. *Am J Cardiol* 1983; **52**: 490–4.

37. Somers VK, Dyken ME, Mark AL, et al. Parasympathetic hyperresponsiveness and bradyarrhythmias during apnea in hypertension. *Clin Auton Res* 1992; **2**: 171–6.

38. Gami AS, Pressman G, Caples SM, et al. Association of atrial fibrillation and obstructive sleep apnea. *Circulation* 2004; **110**: 364–7.

39. Kanagala R, Murali NS, Friedman PA, et al. Obstructive sleep apnea and the recurrence of atrial fibrillation. *Circulation* 2003; **107**: 2589–94.

40. Marsh E, Biller J, Adams H, et al. Circadian variation in onset of acute ischemic stroke. *Arch Neurol* 1990; **47**: 1178–80.

41. Hornyak M, Cejnar M, Elam M, et al. Sympathetic muscle nerve activity during sleep in man. *Brain* 1991; **114**: 1281–95.

42. Somers VK, Dyken ME, Mark AL, et al. Sympathetic nerve activity during sleep in normal humans. *N Engl J Med* 1993; **328**: 303–7.

43. Klingelhofer J, Hajak G, Sander D, et al. Assessment of intracranial hemodynamics in sleep apnea syndrome. *Stroke* 1992; **23**: 1427–33.

44. Jennum P, Borgesen SE. Intracranial pressure and obstructive sleep apnea. *Chest* 1989; **95**: 279–83.

45. Tofler GH, Brezinski D, Schafer AI, et al. Concurrent morning increase in platelet aggregability and the risk of myocardial infarction and sudden cardiac death. *N Engl J Med* 1987; **316**: 1514–18.

46. Fletcher EC, Miller J, Schaaf JW, et al. Urinary catecholamines before and after tracheostomy in patients with obstructive sleep apnea and hypertension. *Sleep* 1987; **10**: 35–44.

47. Geiser T, Buck F, Meyer BJ, et al. In vivo platelet activation is increased during sleep in patients with obstructive sleep apnea syndrome. *Respiration* 2002; **69**: 229–34.

48. Minoguchi K, Yokoe T, Tazaki T, et al. Silent brain infarction and platelet

activation in obstructive sleep apnea. *Am J Respir Crit Care Med* 2007; **175**: 612–17.

49. Iber C, Ancoli-Israel S, Chesson A, et al. *The AASM Manual for the Scoring of Sleep and Associated Events: Rules, Terminology and Technical Specifications*. 1st edn. Westchester, IL: American Academy of Sleep Medicine, 2007.

50. Thomas RJ. Arousals in sleep-disordered breathing: patterns and implications. *Sleep* 2003; **26**: 1042–7.

51. Berry RB, Kouchi KG, Der DE, et al. Sleep apnea impairs the arousal response to airway occlusion. *Chest* 1996; **109**: 1490–6.

52. Cirignotta F, Zucconi M, Mondini S, et al. Cerebral anoxic attacks in sleep apnea syndrome. *Sleep* 1989; **12**: 400–4.

53. Dyken ME, Yamada T, Glenn CL, et al. Obstructive sleep apnea associated with cerebral hypoxemia and death. *Neurology* 2004; **62**: 491–3.

54. White DP, Douglas NJ, Pickett CK, et al. Sleep deprivation and the control of ventilation. *Am Rev Respir Dis* 1983; **198**: 984–6.

55. Issa FG, Sullivan CE. The immediate effects of nasal continuous positive airway pressure treatment on sleep pattern in patients with obstructive sleep apnea syndrome. *Electroencephalogr Clin Neurophysiol* 1986; **63**: 10–17.

56. Sullivan CE, Grunstein RR. Continuous positive airways pressure in sleep-disordered breathing. In: Kryger MH, Roth T, Dement WC, eds. *Principles and Practice of Sleep Medicine*. Philadelphia, PA: Saunders, 1989, 559–70.

57. Berthon-Jones M, Sullivan CE. Ventilation and arousal responses to hypercapnia in normal sleeping humans. *J Appl Physiol* 1984; **57**: 59–67.

58. Buchanan GF, Richerson GB. Central serotonin neurons are required for arousal to CO_2. *Proc Natl Acad Sci U S A* 2010; **107**: 16 354–9.

59. Severson CA, Wang W, Pieribone VA, et al. Midbrain serotonergic neurons are central pH chemoreceptors. *Nat Neurosci* 2003; **6**: 1139–40.

60. Richerson, GB. Serotonergic neurons as carbon dioxide sensors that maintain pH

homeostasis. *Nat Rev Neurosci* 2004; **5**: 449–61.

61. Jouvet M. The role of monoamines and acetylcholine-containing neurons in the regulation of the sleep-waking cycle. *Ergeb Physiol* 1972; **64**: 166–307.

62. Prasad B, Radulovacki M, Olopade C, et al. Prospective trial of efficacy and safety of ondansetron and fluoxetine in patients with obstructive sleep apnea syndrome. *Sleep* 2010; **33**: 982–9.

63. McCann UD, Squambat FP, Swartz AR, et al. Sleep apnea in young abstinent recreational MDMA ("ecstasy") consumers. *Neurology* 2009; **73**: 2011–17.

64. Berthon-Jones M, Sullivan CE. Ventilatory and arousal responses to hypoxia in sleeping humans. *Am Rev Respir Dis* 1982; **125**: 632–9.

65. Darnall RA, Schneider RW, Tobia CM, et al. Arousal from sleep in response to intermittent hypoxia in infant rodents is modulated by medullary raphe GABAergic mechanisms. *Am J Physiol Regul Integr Comp Physiol* 2012; **302**: R551–60.

66. Issa FG, Sullivan CE. Arousal and breathing responses to airway occlusion in healthy sleeping adults. *J Appl Physiol* 1983; **55**: 1113–19.

Sleep apnea and atrial fibrillation

Apoor S. Gami

Introduction

Sleep apnea is associated with several cardiovascular conditions, including arrhythmias [1,2]. Compelling data support a strong relationship between sleep apnea and atrial fibrillation. As industrialized societies contend with burgeoning epidemics of both atrial fibrillation and obesity, understanding this relationship may have important implications for preventing morbidity in individuals and populations.

Epidemiology

Anecdotal recognition of the relationship between sleep apnea and atrial fibrillation has recently given way to more rigorous observational data. The earliest signals were in a 1983 study of 400 middle-aged patients with obstructive sleep apnea who underwent ambulatory electrocardiographic monitoring [3]. The prevalence of nocturnal paroxysmal atrial fibrillation in these patients was greater than 3%, which was five times higher than the expected prevalence of atrial fibrillation in middle-aged community dwellers. Furthermore, in the 12 patients who underwent curative tracheostomy, atrial fibrillation completely resolved by six months.

Later studies noted a high prevalence of sleep apnea in patients with atrial fibrillation. A study of 59 patients with atrial fibrillation but no other cardiovascular conditions found that 32% had polysomnogram-confirmed moderate to severe sleep apnea [4]. Similarly, a high prevalence of atrial fibrillation has been observed in patients with sleep apnea. Analysis of the nocturnal electrocardiographic findings in 566 individuals undergoing polysomnography demonstrated 5% prevalence of atrial fibrillation in those with severe sleep apnea compared to 1% in those without sleep apnea [5]. Another study compared the risk of sleep apnea (based on an internally validated questionnaire) between 151 patients undergoing electrical cardioversion of atrial fibrillation and 463 patients without atrial fibrillation in a cardiology clinic [6]. Despite similar body mass and comorbidities between the groups, the patients with atrial fibrillation had a higher risk of sleep apnea (49%) than the patients without sleep apnea (33%). There was a large, independent association between sleep apnea and atrial fibrillation (odds ratio, 2.2).

Longitudinal observational studies have provided even more compelling data regarding the potential for sleep apnea to indirectly or directly cause atrial fibrillation. A study of 121 patients who underwent polysomnography before coronary artery bypass surgery found that the apnea/hypopnea index and the oxygen desaturation index were both highly predictive of postoperative

---

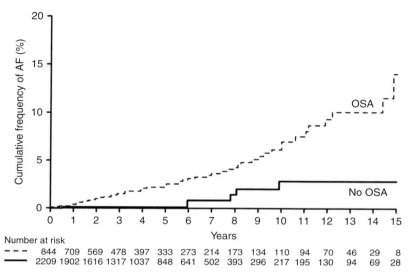

Figure 6.1. The risk of incident (new-onset) atrial fibrillation (AF) in patients with obstructive sleep apnea (OSA) after polysomnography based on the presence or absence of obstructive sleep apnea. (Gami et al. [8], with permission.)

atrial fibrillation [7]. The largest study to assess incident atrial fibrillation evaluated 3542 patients without atrial fibrillation who underwent polysomnography and were followed for an average of five years [8]. In patients younger than 65 years old, nocturnal oxygen desaturation independently and robustly predicted new-onset atrial fibrillation (Figure 6.1).

The risk of recurrence after atrial fibrillation interventions has also been studied longitudinally. An investigation of 106 patients undergoing electrical cardioversion found that after one year, 82% of those with untreated sleep apnea had recurrent atrial fibrillation compared to only 42% of patients with treated sleep apnea and 53% of patients with unknown sleep apnea status [9]. The magnitude and duration of nocturnal oxygen desaturations independently predicted recurrent atrial fibrillation. Several studies have evaluated the effects of sleep apnea on acute and long-term efficacy of atrial fibrillation ablation. In a study of 424 patients undergoing ablation, sleep apnea more than doubled the risk of acute intraprocedural failure [10]. Another study of 3000 patients undergoing ablation found that about 21% had sleep apnea, and that procedural failure was predicted by sleep apnea and noncompliance with continuous positive airway pressure [11]. A meta-analysis of six studies found that polysomnogram-diagnosed sleep apnea increased the risk of recurrent atrial fibrillation after ablation by 40% [12].

Pathophysiology

There are numerous pathophysiological mechanisms that may link sleep apnea to atrial fibrillation (Figure 6.2). One of the most important mechanisms may be the significant changes, both acute and chronic, in autonomic tone that occur with obstructive apneas. Cyclical and simultaneous increases in peripheral sympathetic output and cardiac vagal input occur with each apnea, as do peaks in sympathetic activity with each arousal [13,14]. Negative airway pressure produces cardiac vagal activity that alters atrial conduction

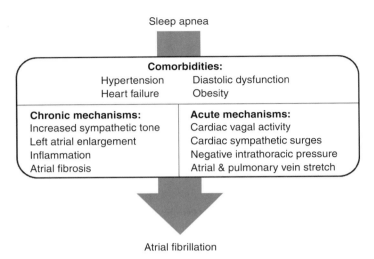

Figure 6.2. The link between sleep apnea and atrial fibrillation may be mediated via multiple comorbidities, and possibly several chronic and acute pathophysiological mechanisms.

properties sufficiently to enhance atrial fibrillation inducibility, a phenomenon that can be prevented by atropine or vagotomy [15]. The sympathetic tone may lead to activation of catecholamine-sensitive ion channel in the atria, which may impact on the frequency of atrial fibrillation triggers. An interventional study in fact showed a higher rate of non-pulmonary vein left atrial triggers during ablation in patients with sleep apnea [11].

Fluctuations in intrathoracic pressure during obstructive apneas may increase cardiac wall stress and atrial stretch [16,17], which can activate stretch-sensitive ion channels or lead to fibrosis at anchoring regions of the atria, such as the pulmonary vein ostium, a site that is critical to atrial fibrillation induction [18].

An important pathophysiological link between sleep apnea and atrial fibrillation is left atrial enlargement. Left atrial size is increased in patients with sleep apnea, perhaps due to associations with hypertension, left ventricular diastolic dysfunction, and obesity. However, it has been shown that in healthy, middle-aged men and women, even when independent of such comorbidities, sleep apnea is associated with increased left atrial size [19]. One potential mechanism may be the cumulative effect of negative intrathoracic pressure during obstructive apneas. In addition, increased systemic inflammation in individuals with sleep apnea may impact on atrial fibrosis, enlargement, and remodeling [20,21]. Atrial electrical remodeling that can contribute to atrial fibrillation maintenance has been demonstrated in interventional studies of patients with sleep apnea, demonstrating reduced atrial voltage, lower atrial conduction time, and widespread increases in complex electrograms [22].

Management

Whether treating sleep apnea directly affects the incidence or frequency of atrial fibrillation has never been rigorously studied in a clinical trial. Confounding factors, such as changes in sleepiness, weight, blood pressure, and lack of patient blinding, would make such a trial difficult to conduct and interpret. Most observational data, however, suggest that the success rates of atrial fibrillation interventions, such as cardioversions and ablation, are significantly improved for patients whose sleep apnea is treated [9,11]. In some individuals a single night of untreated sleep apnea may be enough to precipitate a nocturnal atrial fibrillation recurrence; in others a cumulative effect of untreated sleep apnea may lead to acute intervention failures or subsequent recurrences. The anecdotal experiences of cardiologists challenged with treating atrial fibrillation in the setting of sleep apnea lead most to require that sleep apnea be optimally managed before embarking on specific atrial fibrillation interventions.

Conclusions

A strong relationship exists between sleep apnea and atrial fibrillation. There are numerous plausible pathophysiological mechanisms linking the two, and it is conceivable that some may be causative in given individuals. Epidemiological studies suggest that sleep apnea is a risk factor for new-onset atrial fibrillation, and that its presence reflects a poorer prognosis after atrial fibrillation interventions. Randomized controlled trials are necessary to clarify the effects of sleep apnea therapy on atrial fibrillation outcomes in individuals and communities.

References

1. Gami AS, Caple SM, Somers VK. Sleep-disordered breathing and arrhythmias. In: Zipes DP, Jalife J, eds. *Cardiac Electrophysiology: From Cell to Bedside.* 5th edn. Philadelphia, PA: Saunders, 2009.

2. Gami AS, Somers VK. Sleep apnea and cardiovascular disease. In: Zipes DP, ed. *Braunwald's Heart Disease: A Textbook of Cardiovascular Medicine.* Philadelphia, PA: Saunders, 2007.

3. Guilleminault C, Conolly SJ, Winkle RA. Cardiac arrhythmia and conduction disturbances during sleep in 400 patients with sleep apnea syndrome. *Am J Cardiol* 1983; **52**: 490–4.

4. Porthan KM, Melin JH, Kupila JT, et al. Prevalence of sleep apnea syndrome in lone atrial fibrillation: a case-control study. *Chest* 2004; **125**: 879–85.

5. Mehra R, Benjamin EJ, Shahar E, et al. Association of nocturnal arrhythmias with sleep-disordered breathing: the Sleep Heart Health Study. *Am J Respir Crit Care Med* 2006; **173**: 910–16.

6. Gami AS, Pressman G, Caples SM, et al. Association of atrial fibrillation and obstructive sleep apnea. *Circulation* 2004; **110**: 364–7.

7. Mooe T, Gullsby S, Rabben T, et al. Sleep-disordered breathing: a novel predictor of atrial fibrillation after coronary artery bypass surgery. *Coron Artery Dis* 1996; **7**: 475–8.

8. Gami AS, Hodge DO, Herges RM, et al. Obstructive sleep apnea, obesity, and the risk of incident atrial fibrillation. *J Am Coll Cardiol* 2007; **49**: 565–71.

9. Kanagala R, Murali NS, Friedman PA, et al. Obstructive sleep apnea and the recurrence of atrial fibrillation. *Circulation* 2003; **107**: 2589–94.

10. Sauer WH, McKernan ML, Lin D, et al. Clinical predictors and outcomes associated with acute return of pulmonary vein conduction during pulmonary vein isolation for treatment of atrial fibrillation. *Heart Rhythm* 2006; **3**: 1024–8.

11. Patel D, Mohanty P, Di Biase L, et al. Safety and efficacy of pulmonary vein antral isolation in patients with obstructive sleep apnea: the impact of continuous positive airway pressure. *Circ Arrhythm Electrophysiol* 2010; **3**: 445–51.

12. Ng CY, Liu T, Shehata M, et al. Meta-analysis of obstructive sleep apnea as predictor of atrial fibrillation recurrence after catheter ablation. *Am J Cardiol* 2011; **108**: 47–51.

13. Somers VK, Dyken ME, Clary MP, et al. Sympathetic neural mechanisms in obstructive sleep apnea. *J Clin Invest* 1995; **96**: 1897–904.

14. Somers VK, Dyken ME, Skinner JL. Autonomic and hemodynamic responses and interactions during the Mueller

maneuver in humans. *J Auton Nerv Syst* 1993; **44**: 253–9.

15. Linz D, Schotten U, Neuberger HR, et al. Negative tracheal pressure during obstructive respiratory events promotes atrial fibrillation by vagal activation. *Heart Rhythm* 2011; **8**: 1436–43.

16. Virolainen J, Ventila M, Turto H, et al. Effect of negative intrathoracic pressure on left ventricular pressure dynamics and relaxation. *J Appl Physiol* 1995; **79**: 455–60.

17. Virolainen J, Ventila M, Turto H, et al. Influence of negative intrathoracic pressure on right atrial and systemic venous dynamics. *Eur Heart J* 1995; **16**: 1293–9.

18. Chang SL, Chen YC, Chen YJ, et al. Mechanoelectrical feedback regulates the arrhythmogenic activity of pulmonary veins. *Heart* 2007; **93**: 82–8.

19. Otto ME, Belohlavek M, Romero-Corral A, et al. Comparison of cardiac structural and functional changes in obese otherwise healthy adults with versus without obstructive sleep apnea. *Am J Cardiol* 2007; **99**: 1298–302.

20. Chung M, Martin D, Sprecher D, et al. C-reactive protein elevation in patients with atrial arrhythmias: inflammatory mechanisms and persistence of atrial fibrillation. *Circulation* 2001; **104**: 2886–91.

21. Shamsuzzaman AS, Winnicki M, Lanfranchi P, et al. Elevated C-reactive protein in patients with obstructive sleep apnea. *Circulation* 2002; **105**: 2462–4.

22. Dimitri H, Ng M, Brooks AG, et al. Atrial remodeling in obstructive sleep apnea: implications for atrial fibrillation. *Heart Rhythm* 2012; **9**: 321–7.

Patent foramen ovale, obstructive sleep apnea, and its association with ischemic stroke

Alejandro M. Forteza

Introduction

The advent of diagnostic modalities like transesophageal echocardiography and transcranial Doppler sonography has made the once considered uncommon diagnosis of paradoxical embolism now a rather common and important cause of systemic embolism.

The term paradoxical embolism was first used by Conheim in 1877 to describe venous emboli reaching the systemic arterial circulation through a patent foramen ovale (PFO) [1]. The diagnosis was rarely attempted until noninvasive (or minimally invasive) technology like contrast enhanced echocardiography, transesophageal echocardiography, and transcranial Doppler made it much easier and also shed light on its true incidence. Currently, transesophageal echocardiography is probably the gold standard for the diagnosis of right-to-left intracardiac shunts, and less reliably, intrapulmonary shunts [2–7].

Among the conditions that cause paradoxical embolism, the communications between the atria are the most frequent; the most common of the atrial communications is the PFO. Unfortunately, the working definitions of clinical studies of PFO are extremely variable, and it is possible that several types of intracardiac and intrapulmonary shunts are included in the mostly noninvasive studies.

Embryologically, the common atrium begins to divide into right and left atria in the fifth week of gestation [8]. A membrane, the septum primum, grows caudally from above, fusing with the endocardial cushion and closing a gap known as the ostium primum. From partial resorption of the septum primum, a small defect named the ostium secundum forms. Another septum, the septum secundum, grows from the superior aspect of the common atrium, descending on the right of the septum primum and incompletely covering the ostium secundum. The foramen ovale therefore consists of the incomplete fusion of the septum primum and septum secundum that leaves a cave- or tunnel-like opening that allows oxygenated blood to bypass the lungs during intrauterine life [8] (Figure 7.1).

A high resistance in the collapsed fetal pulmonary circulation increases the arterial blood shunted through the PFO into the left atrium and into the systemic circulation, preferentially to the cerebral and coronary circulation. In most people the PFO closes completely in the first years after birth. This is facilitated by the change in cardiac pressures in the breathing newborn infant. As the resistance in the lungs drops, the right atrial pressure becomes lower than that of the left atrium, leading to a tight contact between the septum primum and secundum, and eventual occlusion of the foramen ovale. Nevertheless, an autopsy study widely quoted found a PFO in 30% of 956 patients with normal hearts [9]. Furthermore, the authors

Sleep, Stroke, and Cardiovascular Disease, ed. Antonio Culebras. Published by Cambridge University Press. © Cambridge University Press 2013.

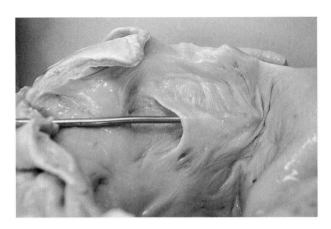

Figure 7.1. Patent foramen ovale; left atrial view. (Photograph courtesy of and reproduced with permission from S Mackey and Jesse E Edwards, Registry for Cardiovascular Disease, St Paul, MN, USA.)

found an incidence of PFO that declined with age: 35% in the first three decades, 25% from the fourth to eighth decades, and falling to 20% in ninth and tenth decades. In addition, the size of the PFO seemed to be larger in older patients [9].These findings suggest that PFOs are very common, even in the older population, and that they continue to close as one gets older.

The high prevalence of PFO has been confirmed by numerous studies, and it is estimated to be within 10%–30% for the general population [10–12], depending on the diagnostic method used.

Association of patent foramen ovale with ischemic stroke

A PFO has been classed as a contributing factor in numerous disease processes. In most of them, the PFO would facilitate a paradoxical embolus or have a thrombus formed *in situ*, causing an arterial occlusion. However, not all embolic material is likely to be thrombus.

Associations have been described with ischemic stroke and more specifically with cryptogenic stroke [13–17]. Cryptogenic stroke is defined as a stroke in which a cause cannot be found despite a thorough and appropriate investigation. Even though the numbers vary, and one could say that there are fewer strokes of unknown origin for the savvy diagnostician, about 40% of all ischemic strokes are classified as cryptogenic by large stroke registries [18]. Lechat et al. reported, in 1988, a small series of 60 adults younger than 55 years of age with ischemic stroke but a normal cardiac examination. They compared these patients with 100 controls, and used transthoracic echocardiography with agitated saline to diagnose PFO in both groups. They found a prevalence of 40% of PFO in the stroke patients and only 10% in the control group (P<0.001). When the stroke patients were analyzed alone, the prevalence of PFO was 21% in 19 patients with an identifiable cause for their stroke; 40% in 15 patients with no identifiable cause but a risk factor for stroke, such as mitral valve prolapse, migraine, or use of contraceptive agents; and 54% in 26 patients with no identifiable cause [14].

In a similar report from New Zealand, Webster et al. studied the prevalence of PFO in patients under the age of 40 years presenting with ischemic stroke or transient ischemic attacks. Patent foramen ovale was diagnosed by contrast echocardiography at rest and with a Valsalva maneuver. Forty stroke patients were enrolled and matched by age and gender to a control group. Right-to-left shunting was found in 20 (50%) of the stroke patients and 6 (15%) of the controls (P<0.001) [13].

These studies, more than proving a relationship, stimulated a myriad of subsequent projects throughout the world. A meta-analysis of nine case-control studies reported just two years later [16] confirmed the association and suggested that young stroke patients have an odds ratio of 3.1 for having a PFO.

More recently, Handke et al. reported a study in which the presence of a PFO was independently associated with cryptogenic stroke in both younger and older patients. In their prospective study, 503 consecutive stroke patients were examined; two hundred and twenty-seven patients were estimated to have a cryptogenic stroke and were compared with the 276 control group of patients with stroke of known cause. All patients underwent transesophageal echocardiography and were examined for the presence of PFO and/or atrial septal aneurysm. A comparison was also made between the 131 patients younger than 55 years of age and the 372 older patients. The prevalence of PFO was greater in patients with cryptogenic stroke than in patients with stroke of a known cause; and this was apparent for both groups, the younger (43.9% vs. 14.3%) and the older (28.3% vs. 11.9%). An even stronger association was observed with PFO plus atrial septal aneurysm and cryptogenic stroke compared to stroke of a known cause in both the younger and the older populations [19]. Nevertheless, controversy still exists and many stroke specialists do not believe in an association between PFO and cryptogenic stroke in the general population [20,21]. Kent et al. argued that by applying Bayes theorem in up to 30% of stroke cases attributed to a PFO, this could just be an incidental finding [21].

If patent foramen ovale is associated with ischemic stroke, how does a patent foramen ovale cause or facilitate a stroke?

The mechanism by which PFOs are associated with ischemic stroke is believed to be para-doxical embolism. In a 20-year natural history study of 2000 consecutive patients, Hutchinson and Acheson reported paradoxical embolism through a PFO as the cause of the stroke in about 4% of their patients, and confirmed their estimate in over 600 autopsies [22]. It is assumed that a venous source, generally undetected, has served as the "clot donor." There are also indications that clots may form directly *in situ*, at the tunnel of the foramen ovale (lurking clot theory) or in its commonly associated atrial septal aneurysm [23].

Shunting through a PFO (blood going from the right atrium to the left atrium) increases with normal physiological Valsalva maneuvers, such as coughing, straining during defecation, lifting weights, or playing certain musical instruments. Increased shunting may also occur in chronic conditions such as chronic obstructive pulmonary disease (COPD), pulmonary hypertension and fibrosis, and any condition that causes a relative increase in right atrial pressures; such is also the case for obstructive sleep apnea (OSA). Finding the venous source of clot remains elusive in most cases, but there is an association among pelvic and lower extremity venous thrombosis and cryptogenic strokes and PFOs. A recent study found that the incidence of pelvic deep vein thrombosis was significantly higher in patients with cryptogenic stroke (20%) and in patients with cryptogenic stroke and PFO (22%), than in patients with stroke of known origin (4%; P<0.025) [24]. The prevalence of PFO was 61% in the cryptogenic stroke population and 19% in the group with stroke of known etiology. The finding that most patients with cryptogenic stroke and pelvic deep vein thrombosis also had a PFO strongly argues in favor of paradoxical embolism as the stroke mechanism. Nevertheless, this has not been agreed by all and controversy still exists.

Atrial arrhythmias, including atrial fibrillation, and a higher atrial vulnerability (threshold electrophysiological stimulus that induces atrial fibrillation for 60 s) are both more commonly observed in patients with PFO, and clearly they could be related to its emboligenic potential [25].

Inherited prothrombotic disorders have also been linked to PFO and stroke. Two studies have found a higher than expected association between ischemic stroke PFO patients and the two most common prothrombotic gene mutations: the prothrombin gene G20210A mutation and the factor V Leiden gene mutation [26,27]. In a separate study, the association with the prothrombin gene mutation was confirmed, but no association was observed with the factor V Leiden gene mutation (the strongest genetic cause of deep vein thrombosis), casting doubts about paradoxical embolism being the mechanism of stroke in patients with PFO [28].

In conclusion one can say that:

- There is overwhelming data supporting the association between PFO and cryptogenic stroke.
- This may be at least more obvious in, but not limited to, young people.
- The most likely mechanism is paradoxical embolism, and other conditions such as acute or chronic elevation of right-sided cardiac pressures, hypercoagulability, and emboligenic cardiac arrhythmias may also contribute.

Decompressive illness

In decompressive illness, nitrogen gaseous bubbles are paradoxically embolized [29,30]. During diving, as the pressure increases according to the depth of the dive, nitrogen breathed in the air becomes dissolved in the blood. During the diver's ascent, the pressure declines, allowing for the formation of nitrogen bubbles, generally in the slower circulating venous blood. These are normally transported to the lungs and exhaled.

In a study performed at Duke University, Durham, NC and published in 1989, 30 patients with a history of decompression sickness were evaluated for a PFO with contrast enhanced echocardiography. Eleven patients (37%) were found to have spontaneous shunting of atrial blood from right-to-left, and 61% of a subgroup with severe diving accidents had shunting compared to only 5% of 176 healthy volunteers [29].

An intracardiac shunt like a PFO has been found to increase the risk of decompression illness five times, and there seems to be a bigger risk, the larger the PFO is [30].

Brain MRI asymptomatic signal abnormalities are more common in divers with PFO than in those who do not have this condition [31,32], and PFO closure seems to prevent major decompressive illness as well as the asymptomatic MRI changes [33].

Migraine with aura

It has been observed that people with migraine with aura have a larger than expected concomitant prevalence of PFO compared to people without migraine (54% vs. 24%) [34]. Vasoactive substances like serotonin would bypass the pulmonary circulation and precipitate migraine. It is also a common observation that migraineurs have a higher prevalence of small bright T2 and FLAIR subcortical abnormalities on brain MRI [35]. A recent large study failed to show an effect of PFO closure on migraine [36], but the methodology of the study has been criticized.

Transient global amnesia

Transient global amnesia is considered to have a similar pathophysiology to migraine, and an association with PFO has also been observed [37].

Fat embolism syndrome

Larger and higher numbers of fat globules are able to reach the systemic circulation if a PFO exists. In a prospective study of unselected femur fractures, Forteza et al. [38] found that only patients with a PFO eventually developed the neurological features of the fat embolism syndrome (FES), and that the presence of a PFO and certain features of the embolic particles as measured by TCD on admission were highly predictive of future occurrences of FES. Other studies agree that an association exists and this is an area of promising research.

Myocardial infarction and peripheral embolism (paradoxical embolism)

Observations about peripheral and coronary artery paradoxical embolism have been made in relation to PFO, strengthening the general concept and suggesting it should be taken into account [39–42].

Patients with pulmonary embolism and PFO seem to be at higher risk for in-hospital cerebral and peripheral embolism as well [42,43], presumably by paradoxical embolism.

Hypoxemia (platypnea–orthodeoxia)

If an opening between the atria (PFO) is large enough and there are higher pressures in the right atrium than in the left atrium, clinical symptoms and signs of hypoxemia may develop. In the platypnea–orthodeoxia syndrome there is severe hypoxemia associated with the upright position in patients with a PFO [44–46]. There are studies showing that correcting the shunt will reverse the hypoxemia [46].

Chronic obstructive pulmonary disease

There is a very high prevalence of PFO in patients with chronic obstructive pulmonary disease (COPD) (up to 70%), and patients with COPD and PFO have worse oxygen desaturations than those without PFO [47].

High-altitude pulmonary edema

There are individuals more susceptible to high-altitude pulmonary edema (HAPE) than others [48]. The cause and the difference between these individuals are incompletely understood. The syndrome is characterized by pulmonary hypertension and arterial hypoxemia at high altitude. In a case-control study of 16 HAPE-susceptible participants and 19 mountaineers resistant to this condition (who have had repeated climbs to peaks above 4000 m and no symptoms of HAPE), PFO was four times more frequent in HAPE-susceptible individuals than in people resistant to this condition. In addition, at high altitude HAPE-susceptible people with a large PFO had more severe hypoxemia. These findings suggest that at high altitude, a large PFO contributes to arterial hypoxemia and facilitates HAPE [48].

Cerebral white matter lesions

The possibility of PFOs being a contributing factor to the development of cerebral white matter abnormalities in migraineurs has been mentioned previously. Patent foramen ovale may also play a role in white matter abnormalities in non-migraine patients. In a study of 115 patients with ischemic strokes, multiple logistic regression analysis showed that the coexistence of PFO and atrial septal aneurysm was significantly associated with the degree of white matter lessions [49]. Other studies have confirmed this higher prevalence of white matter lesions and suggest a frontal predominance [50].

Obstructive sleep apnea

Obstructive sleep apnea is a common disorder characterized by abnormal collapse of the pharyngeal airway during sleep, associated with snoring, failed strong inspiratory efforts, frequent arousals from sleep, and excessive daytime sleepiness. Its consequences and prevalence are so important that it has been called a major public health problem [51].

Besides tiredness and cognitive dysfunction, OSA has been implicated in the development, maintenance, and worsening of numerous forms of cardiovascular disease [52].

The mechanisms mediating the association between OSA and cardiovascular disease are multiple and not all completely understood, but they include:

1. Increase in sympathetic activation [53].
2. Blunting of cerebral hemodynamic and vasomotor reactivity that correlate with apneic episodes [54,55].
3. Ischemia of different vascular beds during the nocturnal apneas, especially the brain and heart.
4. Increase of intracranial pressure.
5. Induction of proinflammatory and prothrombotic factors that play a role in the development of atherosclerosis, including endothelial dysfunction, increased C-reactive protein and cytokine expression, elevated morning fibrinogen levels, and decreased fibrinolytic activity. Increased platelet activity and aggregation as well as a higher hematocrit are also seen. With its inherent stress, the apneic episodes cause a rise in the sympathetic tone being an independent risk factor for hypertension. All of these factors may affect ventricular compliance and afterload causing heart failure and cardiac arrhythmias [56]. Silent and symptomatic coronary syndromes and ischemic strokes have all been associated with OSA [57–60].

For several years it has been known that a history of snoring is independently associated with ischemic stroke, and the relative risk of stroke for individuals that snore has been estimated to be between two- and ten-times higher than for non-snorers [61,62], and seems valid for both men and women. This association between snoring and stroke has been confirmed as being independent from other risk factors in large prospective studies for both men and women [58,60].

In the Sleep Heart Health Study, 6424 individuals were examined with polysomnography at home and asked to self-report cardiovascular events [63]. Sleep-disordered breathing had a stronger association with self-reported heart failure and stroke than with self-reported coronary heart disease.

Nevertheless, an association alone does not imply causality, and it has been difficult to establish whether sleep apnea causes strokes or if, after a stroke, there is a higher incidence of sleep disorders. There are some strong indications, however, that the former is more likely. Patients with transient ischemic attacks or very minor strokes have the same incidence of sleep apnea as those with larger strokes, suggesting that the stroke did not cause the sleep apnea [64].

In another study, central apnea but not obstructive sleep apnea was observed to diminish as time after the stroke elapsed, again suggesting that OSA precedes the ischemic stroke [65].

In a further observational cohort study [66], consecutive patients underwent polysomnography and subsequent strokes and deaths were determined as outcomes. The diagnosis of OSA was established on an apnea/hypopnea index of 5 events/h or higher; patients with an apnea/hypopnea index of <5 events/h served as the comparison group. Of the 1022 patients enrolled, 697 (68%) had OSA. In the unadjusted analysis, OSA was associated with stroke or death from any cause (hazard ratio, 2.24; 95% CI, 1.30–3.86; P=0.004). After adjustment for age, gender, race, smoking status, alcohol-consumption status, body-mass index, and the presence or absence of diabetes mellitus, hyperlipidemia, atrial fibrillation, and hypertension, OSA retained a statistically significant association with stroke or death (hazard ratio, 1.97; 95% CI, 1.12–3.48; P=0.01). The authors concluded that OSA significantly increases the risk of stroke and death from any cause, and that this is independent of other common stroke risk factors.

Obstructive sleep apnea and paradoxical embolism

The mechanisms by which OSA increases the risk of ischemic stroke are multiple and all contribute to the ischemic event. As we have seen, atherosclerosis, facilitation of thrombosis, increased adrenergic tone, cardiac compliance impairment and arrhythmias, a poor vasodilatory response of the cerebral vasculature, added to episodic hypoxemia with decreased cerebral perfusion pressure (elevated intracranial pressure at the end of apneic period) may all play an important role. More recently and due to the accumulated knowledge about PFO and its consequences, the possibility that paradoxical embolism through a PFO as the culprit, at least in some of the strokes related to OSA, has emerged.

As early as 1998, Shanoudy et al. [67] reported on the higher prevalence of PFO in OSA patients and speculated about the contribution of PFO to the observed desaturation. In their study, the prevalence of PFO as estimated by transesophageal echocardiography was 69% (n=48) for the OSA patients, and only 17% (n=24) for normal controls.

In a similar study in which transcranial Doppler was the method used for PFO diagnosis, a right-to-left shunt was found in 21 out of 78 patients with OSA (27%) and in 13 out of 89 control patients (15%) [68].

In another small but thought-provoking experiment, Beelke et al. from Genoa [69] recruited 10 consecutive patients with PFO detectable only under the Valsalva maneuver during wakefulness and affected by OSA. A transcranial Doppler with agitated saline test was conducted while the participants were awake and during periods of apnea/hypopnea in nocturnal sleep. Right-to-left shunting was observed in 9 out of 10 patients and happened during obstructive apneas longer than 17 seconds. The number of microembolic signals (gaseous embolism) detected during nocturnal apneas was positively correlated with the number detected during the Valsalva maneuver in wakefulness (P<0.0001).

The small number of patients in these studies does not allow for strong conclusions, but they do suggest that PFO is more prevalent in patients with OSA and that shunting from right-to-left through a PFO increases with nocturnal apneic events, increasing the risk of paradoxical embolism. Similar findings have been observed in patients with COPD and pulmonary hypertension [47]. A larger size of a PFO as estimated by transesophageal echocardiography in patients with OSA has also been correlated with worse nocturnal desaturations [70].

Supporting the role of PFO in worsening the deranged physiology of OSA are reports on improvement of the sleep apnea with endovascular closure of the PFO [71], and suppression of right-to-left shunting through a PFO with continuous positive airway pressure (CPAP) treatment [72].

There is also a clear increase in the prevalence of pulmonary hypertension in patients with OSA [73–76]. Thus, it is easy to see that the conditions that classically facilitate a paradoxical embolism are all present in patients with sleep apnea and PFO.

From the clinical timing of the onset of symptoms of cerebral ischemia, there are also indications about when these factors may be related to OSA and PFO. In a short communication, Ozdemir et al. reported on two patients with symptoms of cerebral ischemia upon awakening that were found to have a PFO and OSA [77]. The authors speculated that together with the prothrombotic changes associated with OSA, a PFO can facilitate paradoxical embolism, and that the combination of the two conditions should be considered in patients with cryptogenic strokes and symptoms upon awakening.

In a retrospective database analysis of the Stroke Prevention and Atherosclerosis Research Centre (SPARC) in London, Ontario, the same group looked at 175 patients with cryptogenic ischemic stroke or transient ischemic attack who were younger than 70 years old (out of 1609 consecutive patients). Fifty-one percent of the patients had a positive transcranial Doppler shunt test suggestive of a PFO and confirmed by the transesophageal echo (TEE) test.

Factors associated with an ischemic event in patients with PFO were:

1. History of deep vein thrombosis or pulmonary embolism. This was more common in the PFO patients (16%), than in non-PFO patients (5%).
2. Recent prolonged travel, or "economy class stroke syndrome"; 13.4% of PFO patients had an event compared to 3.48% without.
3. Valsalva activities preceding the onset of symptoms; 16.8% in the PFO group compared to 6.9% in the non-PFO group.
4. Waking up with stroke symptoms: 17% in PFO patients compared to 5% for non-PFO patients. The authors [78] speculate that OSA, with its inspiratory efforts, decreases intrathoracic pressure, increases venous return and leftward shift of the septum, acting as a Mueller maneuver. However, no sleep disturbances were reported in their study.
5. A history of migraine.

All of these factors were found to be independently and significantly associated in ischemic stroke PFO patients [78].

Finally, a still unpublished study of 339 consecutive stroke patients, presented at the 2011 American Academy of Neurology meeting [79], found that 39% of patients with the combination of OSA and PFO had their symptoms upon awakening, while without the combination, only 26% of patients had an ischemic event upon awakening (OR=2.2; CI, 1.2–3.9; P=0.01).

Conclusions and clinical implications

According to the presented evidence, it becomes clear that the association of PFO and OSA is common, higher than what would be expected by chance. Furthermore, together they may be a stronger risk factor for stroke than each of them individually.

As the risk seems associated with the multiple physiological abnormalities that accompany OSA and facilitated (at least in the paradoxical embolism case) by a PFO, stroke prevention could potentially be achieved by:

• Improving OSA and reducing the right-to-left shunt (i.e., CPAP treatment).
• Antithrombotic therapy.
• Patent foramen ovale closure.

In our opinion, treatments and especially preventive treatments should be guided toward the original cause of the problem; therefore, the most logical step is to aggressively target the sleep apnea with CPAP. This modality has the capability of reversing the physiological abnormalities, potentially decreasing the risk.

Antithrombotic therapy should be given as well, in light of the greater overall cardiovascular risk. All other risk factors should also be treated, including by the institution of a weight-reduction program.

Patent foramen ovale endovascular or surgical closure cannot be generally recommended at this time [80], but it may well be a consideration in selected patients with multiple risk factors and poor response to CPAP.

This is a very exciting area of interaction between several disciplines, and it will take collaboration between specialists to solve the many questions remaining.

References

1. Conheim J. *Handbuch fur Artze und Studierende*. Berlin: Hirschwald, 1877.
2. Meissner I, Whisnant JP, Khandheria BK, et al. Prevalence of potential risk factors for stroke assessed by transesophageal echocardiography and carotid ultrasonography: the SPARC study. Stroke prevention: assessment of risk in a community. *Mayo Clin Proc* 1999; **74**: 862–9.
3. Hamann GF, Schätzer-Klotz D, Fröhlig G, et al. Femoral injection of echo contrast medium may increase the sensitivity of testing for a patent foramen ovale. *Neurology* 1998; **50**: 1423–8.
4. Spencer MP, Moehring MA, Jesurum J, et al. Power m-mode transcranial Doppler for diagnosis of patent foramen ovale and assessing transcatheter closure. *J Neuroimaging* 2004; **14**: 342–9.
5. Serena J, Segura T, Perez-Ayuso MJ, et al. The need to quantify right-to-left shunt in acute ischemic stroke: a case-control study. *Stroke* 1998; **29**: 1322–8.
6. Jauss M, Zanette E. Detection of right-to-left shunt with ultrasound contrast agent and transcranial Doppler sonography. *Cerebrovasc Dis* 2000; **10**: 490–6.
7. Di Tullio M, Sacco RL, Venketasubramanian N, et al. Comparison of diagnostic techniques for the detection of a patent foramen ovale in stroke patients. *Stroke* 1993; **24**: 1020–4.
8. Azarbal B, Tobis J. Interatrial communications, stroke, and migraine headache. *Appl Neurol* 2005; **1**: 22–36.
9. Hagen PT, Scholz DG, Edwards WD, et al. Incidence and size of patent foramen ovale during the first 10 decades of life: an autopsy study of 965 normal hearts. *Mayo Clin Proc* 1984; **59**: 17–20.
10. Fisher DC, Fisher EA, Budd JH, et al. The incidence of patent foramen ovale in 1,000 consecutive patients. A contrast transesophageal echocardiography study. *Chest* 1995; **107**: 1504–9.
11. Penther P. Patent foramen ovale: an anatomical study. Apropos of 500 consecutive autopsies. *Arch Mal Coeur Vaiss* 1994; **87**: 15–21.
12. Lynch JJ, Schuchard GH, Gross CM, et al. Prevalence of right-to-left atrial shunting in a healthy population: detection by Valsalva maneuver contrast echocardiography. *Am J Cardiol* 1984; **53**: 1478–80.
13. Webster MW, Chancellor AM, Smith HJ, et al. Patent foramen ovale in young stroke patients. *Lancet* 1988; **2**: 11–12.
14. Lechat P, Mas JL, Lascault G, et al. Prevalence of patent foramen ovale in patients with stroke. *N Engl J Med* 1988; **318**: 1148–52.
15. Cabanes L. Mas JL, Cohen A, et al. Atrial septal aneurysm and patent foramen ovale as risk factors for cryptogenic stroke in patients less than 55 years of age. A study using transesophageal echocardiography. *Stroke* 1993; **24**: 1865–73.
16. Overell JR, Bone I, Lees KR. Interatrial septal abnormalities and stroke: a meta-analysis of case-control studies. *Neurology* 2000; **55**: 1172–9.

17. Kerut EK, Norfleet WT, Plotnick GD, et al. Patent foramen ovale: a review of associated conditions and the impact of physiological size. *J Am Coll Cardiol* 2001; **38**: 613–23.

18. Sacco RL, Ellenberg JH, Mohr JP, et al. Infarcts of undetermined cause: the NINCDS Stroke Data Bank. *Ann Neurol* 1989; **25**: 382–90.

19. Handke M, Harloff A, Olschewski M, et al. Patent foramen ovale and cryptogenic stroke in older patients. *N Engl J Med* 2007; **357**: 2262–8.

20. Petty GW, Khandheria BK, Meissner I, et al. Population-based study of the relationship between patent foramen ovale and cerebrovascular ischemic events. *Mayo Clin Proc* 2006; **81**: 602–8.

21. Kent DM, Trikalinos TA, Thaler DE, et al. Patent foramen ovale and cryptogenic stroke. *N Engl J Med* 2008; **358**: 1519–20.

22. Hutchinson EC, Acheson EJ. Strokes: natural history, pathology and surgical treatment. Vol. 4. In: John Walton, ed. *Major Problems in Neurology*. Philadelphia, PA: Saunders, 1975.

23. Falk V, Walther T, Krankenberg H, et al. Trapped thrombus in a patent foramen ovale. *Thorac Cardiovasc Surg* 1997; **45**: 90–2.

24. Cramer SC, Rordorf G, Maki JH, et al. Increased pelvic vein thrombi in cryptogenic stroke: results of the paradoxical emboli from large veins in ischemic stroke (PELVIS) study. *Stroke* 2004; **35**: 46–50.

25. Berthet K, Lavergne T, Cohen A, et al. Significant association of atrial vulnerability with atrial septal abnormalities in young patients with ischemic stroke of unknown cause. *Stroke* 2000; **31**: 398–403.

26. Pezzini A, Del Zotto E, Magoni M, et al. Inherited thrombophilic disorders in young adults with ischemic stroke and patent foramen ovale. *Stroke* 2003; **34**: 28–33.

27. Karttunen V, Hiltunen L, Rasi V, et al. Factor V Leiden and prothrombin gene mutation may predispose to paradoxical embolism in subjects with patent foramen ovale. *Blood Coagul Fibrinolysis* 2003; **14**: 261–8.

28. Lichy C, Reuner KH, Buggle F, et al. Prothrombin G20210A mutation, but not factor V Leiden, is a risk factor in patients with persistent foramen ovale and otherwise unexplained cerebral ischemia. *Cerebrovasc Dis* 2003; **16**: 83–7.

29. Moon RE, Camporesi EM, Kisslo JA. Patent foramen ovale and decompression sickness in divers. *Lancet* 1989; **1**: 513–14.

30. Torti SR, Billinger M, Schwerzmann M, et al. Risk of decompression illness among 230 divers in relation to the presence and size of patent foramen ovale. *Eur Heart J* 2004; **25**: 1014–20.

31. Erdem I, Yildiz S, Uzun G, et al. Cerebral white-matter lesions in asymptomatic military divers. *Aviat Space Environ Med* 2009; **80**: 2–4.

32. Gempp E, Sbardella F, Stephant E, et al. Brain MRI signal abnormalities and right-to-left shunting in asymptomatic military divers. *Aviat Space Environ Med* 2010; **81**: 1008–12.

33. Billinger M, Zbinden R, Mordasini R, et al. Patent foramen ovale closure in recreational divers: effect on decompression illness and ischaemic brain lesions during long-term follow-up. *Heart* 2011; **97**: 1932–7.

34. Diener HC, Kurth T, Dodick D. Patent foramen ovale, stroke, and cardiovascular disease in migraine. *Curr Opin Neurol* 2007; **20**: 310–19.

35. Colombo B, Dalla Libera D, Comi G. Brain white matter lesions in migraine: what's the meaning? *Neurol Sci* 2011; **32**: S37–40.

36. Dowson A, Mullen MJ, Peatfield R, et al. Migraine intervention with STARFlex technology (MIST) trial: a prospective, multicenter, double-blind, sham-controlled trial to evaluate the effectiveness of patent foramen ovale closure with STARFlex septal repair implant to resolve refractory migraine headache. *Circulation* 2008; **117**: 1397–404.

37. Klötzsch C, Sliwka U, Berlit P, et al. An increased frequency of patent foramen ovale in patients with transient global amnesia: analysis of 53 consecutive patients. *Arch Neurol* 1996; **53**: 504–8.

38. Forteza AM, Koch S, Campo-Bustillo I, et al. Transcranial Doppler detection of cerebral fat emboli and relation to paradoxical embolism: a pilot study. *Circulation* 2011; **123**: 1947–52.

39. Rigatelli G, Rigatelli G, Rossi P, et al. Normal angiogram in acute coronary syndromes: the underestimated role of alternative substrates of myocardial ischemia. *Int J Cardiovasc Imaging* 2004; **20**: 471–5.

40. Hugl B, Klein-Weigel P, Posch L, et al. Peripheral ischemia caused by paradoxical embolization: an underestimated problem? *Mt Sinai J Med* 2005; **72**: 200–6.

41. Carano N, Agnetti A, Hagler DJ, et al. Acute myocardial infarction in a child: possible pathogenic role of patent foramen ovale associated with heritable thrombophilia. *Pediatrics* 2004; **114**: e255–8.

42. Steuber C, Panzner B, Steuber T, et al. Open foramen ovale in patients with arterial vascular occlusions of the retina and optic nerve. *Ophthalmologe* 1997; **94**: 871–6.

43. Konstantinides S, Geibel A, Kasper W, et al. Patent foramen ovale is an important predictor of adverse outcome in patients with major pulmonary embolism. *Circulation* 1998; **97**: 1946–51.

44. Shnaider H, Shiran A, Lorber A. Right ventricular diastolic dysfunction and patent foramen ovale causing profound cyanosis. *Heart* 2004; **90**: e31.

45. Nagayoshi Y, Toyama K, Kawano H, et al. Platypnea-orthodeoxia syndrome combined with multiple congenital heart anomalies. *Intern Med* 2005; **44**: 453–7.

46. Guérin P, Lambert V, Godart F, et al. Transcatheter closure of patent foramen ovale in patients with platypnea-orthodeoxia: results of a multicentric French registry. *Cardiovasc Intervent Radiol* 2005; **28**: 164–8.

47. Soliman A, Shanoudy H, Liu J, et al. Increased prevalence of patent foramen ovale in patients with severe chronic obstructive pulmonary disease. *J Am Soc Echocardiogr* 1999; **12**: 99–102.

48. Allemann Y, Hutter D, Lipp E, et al. Patent foramen ovale and high-altitude pulmonary edema. *JAMA* 2006; **296**: 2954–8.

49. Ueno Y, Shimada Y, Tanaka R, et al. Patent foramen ovale with atrial septal aneurysm may contribute to white matter lesions in stroke patients. *Cerebrovasc Dis* 2010; **30**: 15–22.

50. Liu JR, Plötz BM, Rohr A, et al. Association of right-to-left shunt with frontal white matter lesions in T2-weighted MR imaging of stroke patients. *Neuroradiology* 2009; **51**: 299–304.

51. Phillipson EA. Sleep apnea: a major public health problem. *N Engl J Med* 1993; **328**: 1271–3.

52. Shamsuzzaman AS, Gersh BJ, Somers VK. Obstructive sleep apnea: implications for cardiac and vascular disease. *JAMA* 2003; **290**: 1906–14.

53. Narkiewicz K, Somers VK. Sympathetic nerve activity in obstructive sleep apnea. *Acta Physiol Scand* 2003; **177**: 385–90.

54. Morgan BJ, Reichmuth KJ, Peppard PE, et al. Effects of sleep-disordered breathing on cerebrovascular regulation: a population-based study. *Am J Respir Crit Care Med* 2010; **182**: 1445–52.

55. Urbano F, Roux F, Schindler J, et al. Impaired cerebral autoregulation in obstructive sleep apnea. *J Appl Physiol* 2008; **105**: 1852–7.

56. Lavie L. Sleep-disordered breathing and cerebrovascular disease: a mechanistic approach. *Neurol Clin* 2005; **23**: 1059–75.

57. Partinen M, Palomäki H. Snoring and cerebral infarction. *Lancet* 1985; **2**: 1325–6.

58. Koskenvuo M, Kaprio J, Telakivi T, et al. Snoring as a risk factor for ischaemic heart disease and stroke in men. *Br Med J (Clin Res Ed)* 1987; **294**: 16–19.

59. Jennum P, Schultz-Larsen K, Davidsen M, et al. Snoring and risk of stroke and ischemic heart disease in a 70 year old population. A 6-year follow up study. *Int J Epidemiol* 1994; **23**: 1159–64.

60. Hu FB, Willett WC, Manson JE, et al. Snoring and risk of cardiovascular disease in women. *J Am Coll Cardiol* 2000; **35**: 308–13.

61. Smirne S, Palazzi S, Zucconi M, et al. Habitual snoring as a risk factor for acute vascular disease. *Eur Respir J* 1993; **6**: 1357–61.

62. Neau JP, Meurice JC, Paquereau J, et al. Habitual snoring as a risk factor for brain infarction. *Acta Neurol Scand* 1995; **92**: 63–8.

63. Shahar E, Whitney CW, Redline S, et al. Sleep-disordered breathing and cardiovascular disease: cross-sectional results of the Sleep Heart Health Study. *Am J Respir Crit Care Med* 2001; **163**: 19–25.

64. Bassetti C, Aldrich MS. Sleep apnea in acute cerebrovascular diseases: final report on 128 patients. *Sleep* 1999; **22**: 217–23.

65. Parra O, Arboix A, Bechich S, et al. Time course of sleep-related breathing disorders in first-ever stroke or transient ischemic attack. *Am J Respir Crit Care Med* 2000; **161**: 375–80.

66. Yaggi HK, Concato J, Kernan WN, et al. Obstructive sleep apnea as a risk factor for stroke and death. *N Engl J Med* 2005; **353**: 2034–41.

67. Shanoudy H, Soliman A, Raggi P, et al. Prevalence of patent foramen ovale and its contribution to hypoxemia in patients with obstructive sleep apnea. *Chest* 1998; **113**: 91–6.

68. Beelke M, Angeli S, Del Sette M, et al. Prevalence of patent foramen ovale in subjects with obstructive sleep apnea: a transcranial Doppler ultrasound study. *Sleep Med* 2003; **4**: 219–23.

69. Beelke M, Angeli S, Del Sette M, et al. Obstructive sleep apnea can be provocative for right-to-left shunting through a patent foramen ovale. *Sleep* 2002; **25**: 856–62.

70. Johansson MC, Eriksson P, Peker Y, et al. The influence of patent foramen ovale on oxygen desaturation in obstructive sleep. *Eur Respir J* 2007; **29**: 149–55.

71. Silver B, Greenbaum A, McCarthy S. Improvement in sleep apnea associated with closure of a patent foramen ovale. *J Clin Sleep Med* 2007; **3**: 295–6.

72. Pinet C, Orehek J. CPAP suppression of awake right-to-left shunting through patent foramen ovale in a patient with obstructive sleep apnea. *Thorax* 2005; **60**: 880–1.

73. Alchanatis M, Paradellis G, Pini H, et al. Left ventricular function in patients with obstructive sleep apnoea syndrome before and after treatment with nasal continuous positive airway pressure. *Respiration* 2000; **67**: 367–71.

74. Laks L, Lehrhaft B, Grunstein RR, et al. Pulmonary hypertension in obstructive sleep apnoea. *Eur Respir J* 1995; **8**: 537–41.

75. Sanner BM, Doberauer C, Konermann M, et al. Pulmonary hypertension in patients with obstructive sleep apnea syndrome. *Arch Intern Med* 1997; **157**: 2483–7.

76. Krieger J, Sforza E, Apprill M, et al. Pulmonary hypertension, hypoxemia, and hypercapnia in obstructive sleep apnea patients. *Chest* 1989; **96**: 729–37.

77. Ozdemir O, Beletsky V, Hachinski V, et al. Cerebrovascular events on awakening, patent foramen ovale and obstructive sleep apnea syndrome. *J Neurol Sci* 2008 ; **268**: 193–4.

78. Ozdemir AO, Tamayo A, Munoz C, et al. Cryptogenic stroke and patent foramen ovale: clinical clues to paradoxical embolism. *J Neurol Sci* 2008; **275**: 121–7.

79. Ciccone A, Nobili L, Roccatagliata DV, et al. Causal role of sleep apneas and patent foramen ovale in wake-up stroke. *Neurology* 2011; **76**: A170.

80. Furlan AJ, Reisman M, Massaro J, et al. Closure or medical therapy for cryptogenic stroke with patent foramen ovale. *N Engl J Med* 2012; **366**: 991–9.

Pathogenesis of cerebral small-vessel disease in obstructive sleep apnea

Gustavo C. Román

Introduction

Elderly women affected by obstructive sleep apnea (OSA) develop cognitive deficits [1] compared to age-matched controls with normal sleep. Yaffe and her colleagues [1] concluded that the cognitive decline correlated with hypoxemia rather than with the fragmentation of the sleep architecture resulting from apneas and hypopneas. A similar deleterious effect of OSA on cognitive function has been demonstrated in patients referred to the Alzheimer and dementia clinic of the Methodist Neurological Institute in Houston, TX (Román, unpublished data). Moreover, in the latter patients, magnetic resonance imaging (MRI) of the brain showed that OSA was accompanied by varying degrees of cerebral small-vessel disease, in particular periventricular hyperintensities of the white matter and lacunar strokes, explaining the clinical picture of subcortical prefrontal dysfunction observed in these patients, in isolation or mixed with features of Alzheimer's disease. In this chapter, the postulated pathogenesis of cerebral small-vessel disease in subjects with OSA is reviewed.

Cognitive and vascular consequences of sleep apnea

Sound sleep is critical for cognitive function, in particular because of its effects on synaptic plasticity and consolidation of memory [2]. Therefore, disruption of sleep and fragmentation of the sleep architecture are detrimental for memory. Moreover, sleep is a vital ancestral need and prolonged sleep deprivation leads to death in several species[2], including humans with fatal familial insomnia, a prion disease[3]. The deleterious effects of OSA on the vascular and circulatory systems are well recognized and include development of hypertension, coronary artery disease, heart failure, myocardial infarction, pulmonary hypertension, atrial fibrillation, stroke, ruptured aortic aneurysms, and sudden cardiac death[4].

Sorajja et al. [5] estimated that as many as 20% of middle-aged adults have mild OSA and 4%–9% exhibit the OSA syndrome with excessive daytime sleepiness. The current epidemic of obesity has substantially increased the population at risk for development of OSA and its consequences, particularly the metabolic syndrome [6,7]. Interestingly, among other factors, obesity has been linked to decreased sleep time in adults [8] and children [9].

Sleep, Stroke, and Cardiovascular Disease, ed. Antonio Culebras. Published by Cambridge University Press. © Cambridge University Press 2013.

Definition and pathogenesis

McNicholas and Javaheri [10] define OSA as a form of periodic breathing occurring during sleep characterized by intermittent episodes of complete or incomplete upper airway occlusion (respectively, apneas and hypopneas). The presence of small-vessel pathology in patients with OSA has seldom been studied. When compared with patients with Alzheimer's disease or with matched controls, patients with multi-infarct dementia had a higher prevalence of OSA [11]. Additionally, OSA has been associated with white matter lesions [12] and lacunar strokes [13]. Small-vessel disease appears to be the result of complex mechanisms (stress-induced, hormonal, and inflammatory) provoked by the apneas and hypopneas.

Inspiration is the result of increased motor activity of respiratory inspiratory muscles. Patency of the upper airway during inspiration is mediated by activation of the pharyngeal dilator muscles. Inspiration begins with activation of rostral pontine respiratory neurons that stimulate firing of cells of the solitary tract nucleus and of other neurons in the dorsal medullary respiratory group, along with cells of the medullary ventral group, particularly in the nucleus ambiguus. Impulses are carried by the phrenic and intercostal nerves, leading to contraction of the diaphragm and intercostal muscles, resulting in expansion of the thoracic cavity. Inspiration concludes when pulmonary stretch afferences stimulate the pontine apneustic center that in turn inhibits medullary inspiratory neurons. The main stimulus for respiratory inspiration is the activation of carotid and aortic body chemoreceptors by a decrease in blood oxygen concentration (SaO_2) and to a lesser extent by an increase in arterial CO_2 and by blood acidosis (lower pH).

Airway obstruction during sleep may result from decreased neural activation of pharyngeal dilator muscles predisposing the airway to collapse [4]. Moreover, a crowded oropharynx, due to adiposity, macroglossia, or enlarged tonsils and adenoids, is an important cause of OSA given that the decrease in lumen diameter increases the airway resistance as a result of Poiseuille's law principles (which states that resistance increases rapidly as diameter decreases); therefore, greater inspiratory negative pressure is required. However, upper airway narrowing is responsible only for the oropharyngeal component of the obstruction in sleep apnea. For this reason, the uvulopalatopharyn-goplasty (UPPP), a common surgical procedure for snoring and OSA, carries a success rate of only 40%.

The most important component of sleep apneas and hypopneas is obstruction of the upper airway by the tongue. The extrinsic muscles of the tongue (genioglossus, genio-hyoid) are inserted on the inner surface of the mandible and as muscle relaxation occurs during non-rapid eye movement (NREM) and REM sleep, the jaw drops and the tongue falls back, blocking the airway. For these reasons, snoring and apneas are worse when patients sleep on their backs (positional apnea) while sleeping on the side improves the snoring and decreases the apneas. Patients with chronic nasal obstruction from allergies or anatomical defects of the nasal septum and turbinates tend to breathe through an open mouth during sleep and are more likely to develop OSA. This mechanism also explains the positive effects on OSA of dental retainers and elastic chin straps that prevent jaw dropping; in more severe cases, surgical treatment may be required using procedures such as mandibular reconstruction (genioglossus advancement), hyoid bone advance-ment, or even maxillomandibular advancement in patients with micrognathia, in order to control severe apneas and hypopneas during sleep.

Table 8.1. Alterations induced by apneas and hypopneas during sleep

1.	Recurrent hypoxemia (low arterial SaO$_2$), hypercapnia (elevated arterial SaCO$_2$), and respiratory acidosis (low blood pH)
2.	Activation of carotid and aortic chemoreceptors
3.	Reflex contractions of respiratory chest and abdominal muscles
4.	Severely increased negative intrathoracic pressure
5.	Tachycardia from atrial Bainbridge reflex
6.	Sympathetic (adrenergic) outburst
7.	Arterial hypertension
8.	Baroreceptor reflex activation
9.	Peripheral vasoconstriction
10.	Hyperglycemia
11.	Hypercoagulability
12.	Repeated arousals and awakenings

SaO$_2$(CO$_2$), arterial oxygen (carbon dioxide) saturation.

Alterations resulting from airway obstruction

Interruption of ventilation as a result of airway obstruction produces repetitive hypoxemia due to a decrease of arterial blood oxygenation (SaO$_2$) of varying duration and severity, accompanied by concomitant carbon dioxide (CO$_2$) retention, with elevation of arterial CO$_2$ or hypercapnia and respiratory acidosis. Intermittent, often violent and strenuous, respiratory efforts occur as a result of reflex attempts involving chest and abdominal musculature to overcome the obstruction of the airway and to restore airflow. These efforts (Mueller maneuver) generate severely negative intrathoracic pressure. The end result of these respiratory events is suffocation that produces an acute stress reaction, disrupts sleep, causes arousal from deep sleep to more superficial sleep stages, and finally awakens the subject, lowering sleep efficiency and reducing total sleep time (Table 8.1). The number of apneas and hypopneas per hour (apnea/hypopnea index, AHI), the degree of oxygen desaturation, and the number of arousals and awakenings per hour constitute the main elements to quantify the severity of OSA.

Cardiac consequences of mechanical changes induced by sleep apnea

The activation of carotid body and aortic chemoreceptors by the hypoxemia of sleep apnea stimulates inspiratory neurons, resulting in the Mueller maneuver or occluded inspiration whereby the diaphragm and respiratory chest muscles continue to exhibit intermittent and violent contractions in a reflex effort to resume ventilation. Negative intrathoracic pressures as low as −60 to −80 mmHg are generated, causing an increase in central venous pressure and atrial distension, leading to reflex tachycardia (Bainbridge reflex), as well as to alterations in cardiac morphology and left ventricular function [4]. The negative intrathoracic pressure assists left ventricular ejection and results in higher left ventricular afterload that eventually leads to structural thickening of the left ventricle wall and diastolic dysfunction [14]. Similar increases in negative transmural pressure affect the atrial wall, resulting in repetitive atrial stretching with eventual left atrial enlargement, reflected by an increased left atrial volume index and alterations of diastolic function that predispose to atrial fibrillation and heart failure [15].

Autonomic and hemodynamic consequences of obstructive sleep apnea

Lurie [16] has recently reviewed the topic of the hemodynamic changes observed in OSA as a result of alterations in the activity of the autonomic nervous system. As mentioned previously, early in the course of an apnea, the heart rate may increase due to the Bainbridge reflex. Simultaneously, the blood pressure decreases at the start of the apnea from baroreceptor activation and vagal (parasympathetic) response; this is followed by a hypertensive response at the terminal portion of the apnea due to sympathetic activation resulting from the acute stress response to suffocation. This response includes release of adrenaline from sympathetic neurons as well as noradrenaline and cortisol from the adrenal medulla and cortex, respectively. Sympathetic activation is even further exacerbated by a potentiated sensitivity of the chemoreflex response to hypoxemia in OSA patients [17]. Sympathetic-mediated vasoconstriction results in increase in blood pressure, particularly at the end of apnea when resumption of breathing increases cardiac output into a vasoconstricted periphery causing an abrupt reduction in left ventricular stroke volume.

In summary, during the very early phase of the apnea, the vagal response suppresses sympathetic nerve activity; the latter then increases and reaches a peak at the end of the apnea and on arousal. When ventilation resumes, sympathetic activity in peripheral blood vessels is inhibited. Ventilation occurs in the context of peripheral vasoconstriction and increased peripheral resistance due to the kinetics of norepinephrine at the neurovascular junction [16]. These hemodynamic responses occur concurrently with severe hypoxemia, hypercapnia, and acidosis imposing severe stress on the cardiac and vascular system [4]. A typical patient with severe OSA may have an AHI of >60 events/h; that is, upward of one apnea per minute. Owing to the constant repetition of this sequence, there is an eventual blunting of the chemoreceptor and baroreceptor reflexes [18], increasing the length of the apneas and the severity of the hypoxemia. The net result is the increased risk of pulmonary hypertension, cardiac arrhythmias, and sudden death.

The mechanisms activated by OSA, in particular the sympathetic hyperactivity, persist during daytime, along with the associated vascular, pulmonary, and endocrine responses [19]. The hypoxemia and sympathetic activation often causes treatment-resistant systemic hypertension along with endothelial dysfunction as manifested by vasoconstriction mediated by elevated plasma endothelin-1 levels [20,21] and decreased plasma levels of the endothelial vasodilator nitrous oxide [22]. It has been shown that the potent vasoconstrictor endothelin increases for several hours with untreated OSA [23] but the levels decrease after treatment with continuous positive airway pressure (CPAP).

Inflammation in sleep apnea

Patients with OSA develop a proinflammatory state evidenced by increased C-reactive protein [24] and increased expression of adhesion molecules and reactive oxygen species in leukocytes [25]. The resultant vasoconstriction, abnormal cell proliferation, and hypercoagulability may initiate or worsen the progression of atherosclerotic cardiovascular disease, stroke, and cerebro-vascular disorders [21]. The repetitive cycles of hypoxemia/reperfusion injury of OSA cause oxidative stress and contribute to endothelial and vascular damage due to production of free radicals [5,26]. For instance, levels of homocysteine–a sulfur-containing amino acid capable of causing endothelial oxidative damage–are often elevated in patients with OSA, particularly those with ischemic heart disease [27–29]. Of interest, CPAP therapy lowers homocysteine levels by about 30% [30].

Metabolic syndrome and sleep apnea

Obesity and the metabolic syndrome frequently occur in patients with OSA. These patients often have glucose intolerance [31] and diabetes [32] due to insulin resistance, obesity [33], and elevated leptin levels. Leptin is produced by the adipocyte and is strongly associated with obesity; of interest, leptin may modulate the central control of ventilatory mechanisms, particularly in patients with congestive heart failure [34].

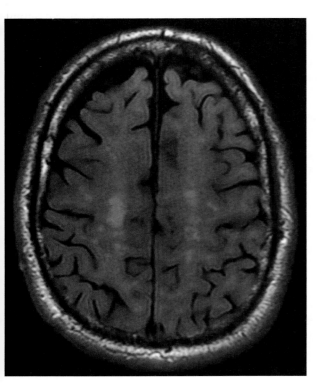

Figure 8.1. Brain MRI, coronal FLAIR image, demonstrating numerous lacunar lesions in the subcortical white matter in a male patient, 83 years old, with a history of mild cognitive impairment of the amnestic/dysexecutive type and chronic rhinitis with turbinate hypertrophy. Polysomnography demonstrated obstructive sleep apnea with low sleep efficiency at 70%, decreased rapid eye movement (REM) sleep and slow-wave sleep percentages (5.4% and 0.3%, respectively), with a long latency to REM sleep at 103 minutes. The apnea/hypopnea index was 20 events/h and the oxygen saturation nadir was 82%.

Thrombosis

Normally, the "flight or fight" response (acute stress reaction) is accompanied by increased coagulation. It is not surprising then that patients with OSA exhibit increased fibrinogen, hematocrit, plasminogen activator inhibitor-1, and platelet aggregability [4]. In severe cases of OSA, chronic hypoxemia leads to stimulation of erythropoietin and development of polycythemia. Moreover, as mentioned earlier, the presence of inflammatory mediators such as adhesion molecules and cytokines contribute to leukocyte adhesion, endothelial damage, and hence to thrombosis and atherosclerosis.

Conclusion

Obstructive sleep apnea is a common contemporary problem linked to obesity and the metabolic syndrome. Obstructive sleep apnea is a well-recognized cause of the most severe vascular risk factors leading to stroke and ischemic heart disease. It has been recognized only recently that OSA also leads to cognitive dysfunction not only as a result of sleep disruption but more likely from the effects of chronic hypoxia and sympathetic stress causing small-vessel disease in the brain, white matter ischemia, and lacunar strokes (Figure 8.1). It is hoped that early recognition and treatment with CPAP will result in improvement of cognitive function [35] and prevention of dementia.

References

1. Yaffe K, Laffan AM, Harrison SL, et al. Sleep-disordered breathing, hypoxia, and risk of mild cognitive impairment and dementia in older women. *JAMA* 2011; **306**: 613–19.

2. Wang G, Grone B, Colas D, et al. Synaptic plasticity in sleep: learning, homeostasis and disease. *Trends Neurosci* 2011; **34**: 452–63.

3. Fiorino AS. Sleep, genes and death: fatal familial insomnia. *Brain Res Brain Res Rev* 1996; **22**: 258–64.

4. Lopez-Jimenez F, Kuniyoshi FHS, Gami A, et al. Obstructive sleep apnea: implications for cardiac and vascular disease. *Chest* 2008; **133**: 793–804.

5. Sorajja D, Gami AS, Somers VK, et al. Independent association between obstructive sleep apnea and subclinical coronary artery disease. *Chest* 2008; **133**: 927–33.

6. Batsis JA, Nieto-Martinez RE, Lopez-Jimenez F. Metabolic syndrome: from global epidemiology to individualized medicine. *Clin Pharmacol Ther* 2007; **82**: 509–24.

7. Reaven GM. Insulin resistance: the link between obesity and cardiovascular disease. *Med Clin North Am* 2011; **95**: 875–92.

8. Vorona RD, Winn MP, Babineau TW, et al. Overweight and obese patients in a primary care population report less sleep than patients with a normal body mass index. *Arch Intern Med* 2005; **165**: 25–30.

9. Sekine M, Yamagami T, Handa K, et al. A dose-response relationship between short sleeping hours and childhood obesity: results of the Toyama Birth Cohort Study. *Child Care Health Dev* 2002; **28**: 163–70.

10. McNicholas WT, Javaheri S. Pathophysiologic mechanisms of cardiovascular disease in obstructive sleep apnea. *Sleep Med Clin* 2007; **2**: 539–47.

11. Erkinjuntti T, Partinen M, Sulkava R, et al. Sleep apnea in multi-infarct dementia and Alzheimer's disease. *Sleep* 1987; **10**: 419–25.

12. Harbison J, Birchall D, Zammit-Maempell I, et al. White matter disease and sleep-disordered breathing after acute stroke. *Neurology* 2003; **61**: 959–63.

13. Bassetti CL, Milanova M, Gugger M. Sleep-disordered breathing and acute ischemic stroke: diagnosis, risk factors, treatment, evolution, and long-term clinical outcome. *Stroke* 2006; **37**: 967–72.

14. Arias MA, Garcia-Rio F, Alonso-Fernandez A, et al. Obstructive sleep apnea syndrome affects left ventricular diastolic function:

effects of nasal continuous positive airway pressure in men. *Circulation* 2005; **112**: 375–83.

15. Otto ME, Belohlavek M, Romero-Corral A, et al. Comparison of cardiac structural and functional changes in obese otherwise healthy adults with versus without obstructive sleep apnea. *Am J Cardiol* 2007; **99**: 1298–302.

16. Lurie A. Hemodynamic and autonomic changes in adults with obstructive sleep apnea. *Adv Cardiol* 2011; **46**: 171–95.

17. Narkiewicz K, van de Borne PJ, Montano N, et al. Contribution of tonic chemoreflex activation to sympathetic activity and blood pressure in patients with obstructive sleep apnea. *Circulation* 1998; **97**: 943–5.

18. Grassi G, Seravalle G, Quarti-Trevano F, et al. Reinforcement of the adrenergic overdrive in the metabolic syndrome complicated by obstructive sleep apnea. *J Hypertens* 2010; **28**: 1313–20.

19. Lopez-Jimenez F, Somers VK. Stress measures linking sleep apnea, hypertension and diabetes - AHI vs arousals vs hypoxemia. *Sleep* 2006; **29**: 743–4.

20. Phillips BG, Narkiewicz K, Pesek CA, et al. Effects of obstructive sleep apnea on endothelin-1 and blood pressure. *J Hypertens* 1999; **17**: 61–6.

21. Karkoulias K, Lykouras D, Sampsonas F, et al. The role of endothelin-1 in obstructive sleep apnea syndrome and pulmonary arterial hypertension: pathogenesis and endothelin-1 antagonists. *Curr Med Chem* 2010; **17**: 1059–66.

22. Schulz R, Schmidt D, Blum A, et al. Decreased plasma levels of nitric oxide derivatives in obstructive sleep apnoea: response to CPAP therapy. *Thorax* 2000; **55**: 1046–51.

23. Allahdadi KJ, Walker BR, Kanagy NL. Augmented endothelin vasoconstriction in intermittent hypoxia-induced hypertension. *Hypertension* 2005; **45**: 705–7.

24. Shamsuzzaman AS, Winnicki M, Lanfranchi P, et al. Elevated C-reactive protein in patients with obstructive sleep apnea. *Circulation* 2002; **105**: 2462–4.

25. Dyugovskaya L, Lavie P, Lavie L. Increased adhesion molecules expression and production of reactive oxygen species in leukocytes of sleep apnea patients. *Am J Respir Crit Care Med* 2002; **165**: 934–9.

26. Suzuki YJ, Jain V, Park AM, et al. Oxidative stress and oxidant signaling in obstructive sleep apnea and associated cardiovascular diseases. *Free Radic Biol Med* 2006; **40**: 1683–92.

27. Lavie L, Perelman A, Lavie P. Plasma homocysteine levels in obstructive sleep apnea. Association with cardiovascular morbidity. *Chest* 2001; **120**: 900–8.

28. Svatikova A, Wolk R, Magera MJ, et al. Plasma homocysteine in obstructive sleep apnoea. *Eur Heart J* 2004; **25**: 1325–9.

29. Winnicki M, Palatini P. Obstructive sleep apnoea and plasma homocysteine: an overview. *Eur Heart J* 2004; **25**: 1281–3.

30. Jordan W, Berger C, Cohrs S, et al. CPAP-therapy effectively lowers serum homocysteine in obstructive sleep apnea syndrome. *J Neural Transm* 2004; **111**: 683–9.

31. Sulit L, Storfer-Isser A, Kirchner HL, et al. Differences in polysomnography predictors for hypertension and impaired glucose tolerance. *Sleep* 2006; **29**: 777–83.

32. Reichmuth KJ, Austin D, Skatrud JB, et al. Association of sleep apnea and type II diabetes: a population-based study. *Am J Respir Crit Care Med* 2005; **172**: 1590–5.

33. Phillips BG, Kato M, Narkiewicz K, et al. Increases in leptin levels, sympathetic drive, and weight gain in obstructive sleep apnea. *Am J Physiol Heart Circ Physiol* 2000; **279**: H234–7.

34. Wolk R, Johnson BD, Somers VK. Leptin and the ventilator response to exercise in heart failure. *J Am Coll Cardiol* 2003; **42**: 1644–9.

35. Matthews EE, Aloia MS. Cognitive recovery following positive airway pressure (PAP) in sleep apnea. *Prog Brain Res* 2011; **190**: 71–88.

Sleep apnea and acute stroke deterioration

Kristian Barlinn and Andrei V. Alexandrov

Synopsis

Sleep-disordered breathing of variable degrees is associated with an increased risk of neurological deterioration within the first 72 hours after stroke onset. The pathogenic link between sleep apnea and acute deterioration in ischemic stroke patients is now a subject of clinical investigations. Vasomotor reactivity and intracranial blood flow steal in response to changing vasodilatory stimuli like carbon dioxide play a pivotal role in clinical deterioration with reversed Robin Hood syndrome. A mechanical ventilatory correction in acute stroke patients might have a beneficial effect on sleep apnea and brain perfusion. This is a novel therapeutic target and the missing link in the pathogenesis of early neurological deterioration and stroke recurrence.

This chapter reviews the present knowledge of sleep-disordered breathing and acute neurological deterioration in stroke patients, highlighting clinical studies addressing this issue, and discusses future directions regarding noninvasive ventilatory correction to reverse cerebral blood flow (CBF) steal or even to augment blood flow in these patients. We cover sleep-disordered breathing and its acute assessment for non-sleep-disorder readers, ultrasound and hemodynamics for all readers, and specific steps that stroke specialists can currently make to identify these patients and possibly treat them early.

Acute stroke deterioration

Numerous terms and a variety of definitions have been used in the literature to describe the condition of clinical deterioration in acute and subacute phases after a stroke [1–6]. Regardless of the particular definition used, it implies a gradual or stepwise worsening of the neurological deficit, usually measured by a structured neurological scale such as the National Institutes of Health Stroke Scale (NIHSS) score. Deterioration occurs after a temporary stabilization or even improvement from the initial stroke severity, either at the time of symptom onset or on admission to the hospital. What degree of neurological deterioration should prompt emergent change in management remains controversial. The European Cooperative Acute Stroke Study investigators diagnosed neurological deterioration when there was a decrease of ≥2 points in consciousness or motor function; the Scandinavian Neurological Stroke Scale used a decrease of ≥3 points in speech function between the day of admission and day seven [6], while the Canadian Neurological Scale used a decrease of ≥1 point [7]. However, the NIHSS score is the most widely used scoring system

Sleep, Stroke, and Cardiovascular Disease, ed. Antonio Culebras. Published by Cambridge University Press. © Cambridge University Press 2013.

to assess neurological deficits in clinical trials; thus, we favor an increase in the NIHSS score by two or more points (or stroke-related death) between admission and day five of hospitalization as the criterion for acute stroke deterioration [1]. Of note, this definition is significantly associated with worse outcomes in acute stroke patients [1].

Depending on clinical definitions, underlying pathophysiology, and time of admission to the hospital, acute stroke deterioration is estimated to occur in between one and two of five patients with acute ischemic stroke [5,8,9]. Although various and heterogeneous causes of acute stroke deterioration have been proposed, there is general agreement that it occurs most commonly in patients with hemorrhagic strokes followed by noncardioembolic strokes and least frequently in patients with cardioembolic ischemic strokes. According to subtypes of ischemic strokes, patients with lacunar infarcts and large-artery occlusive disease seem at risk of neurological deterioration with rates of 37% and 33%, respectively [8]. Moreover, symptomatic intracranial atherosclerotic disease (IAD) has been implicated in the pathophysiology of neurological deterioration during hospitalization. Even though different definitions for neurological deterioration were used in two recent studies, about 15% of acute stroke patients with IAD deteriorated acutely during its clinical course [10,11].

We summarize independent clinical and radiological predictors of acute stroke deterioration in Table 9.1 [4,12–24].

Sleep apnea as predictor of acute stroke deterioration

Long-recognized mechanisms of acute stroke deterioration (Table 9.1) do not account for all cases of neurological deterioration or symptom recurrence. Several studies have provided evidence that sleep apnea of a variable degree is an independent risk factor for stroke (particularly ischemic stroke), which is similar in clinical significance to that of other well-established vascular risk factors [25,26]. A prospective cohort study found that obstructive sleep apnea (OSA) increases the risk for stroke and death from any cause by almost two-fold and independently of other vascular risk factors (hazard ratio, 1.97; 95% CI, 1.1–3.5) [26]. Following stroke, sleep apnea negatively affects length of hospitalization, short-term as well as long-term outcome, and further increases the risk of stroke recurrence [27]. Moreover, sleep apnea has been associated with an increased risk of neurological deterioration within the first 72 hours after stroke onset [24].

In a prospective study by Iranzo and colleagues, 50 acute ischemic stroke patients underwent all-night polysomnography (PSG) in the first night after stroke onset and were followed up for six months [24]. Early neurological deterioration was defined as a decrease of at least two points in the Scandinavian Stroke Scale score between admission and day three of hospitalization. Sleep apnea, defined as an AHI of ≥10 events/h, was present in 31 (62%) patients (OSA in 30%) and early neurological deterioration was detected in 15 (30%) patients. Early neurological deterioration within the first days after stroke onset was independently predicted by sleep apnea (OR 8.2; 95% CI, 1.3–51.2) and was associated with worse functional outcome at discharge (P<0.001). The authors speculated that early neurological worsening reflects neuronal damage within the ischemic penumbra due to hemodynamic disturbances during apnea episodes. However, before discussing potential pathogenic mechanisms that account for neurological deterioration in patients with acute ischemic stroke and sleep apnea, it is important to recapitulate systemic and cerebral hemodynamic principles.

Table 9.1. Potential independent predictors of acute stroke deterioration during hospitalization (we do not separate the time points when deterioration may occur–early, late or both). Some of these predictors are mutually dependent.

Independent predictors of acute stroke deterioration	
Clinical	**Imaging**
Older age	Computed tomography
Stroke severity on admission • e.g., NIHSS >7 points	• Hyperdense MCA sign • >1/3 MCA infarctions • Cerebral edema • Large perfusion deficit (on CTP)
Subtype of stroke	Magnetic resonance imaging
• Intracerebral hemorrhage • Posterior circulation strokes • Non-cardioembolic > cardioembolic ischemic strokes • Lacunar > non-lacunar infarctions	• Large DWI lesions • Large PWI lesions
Blood pressure	CT- or MR-angiography
• Arterial hypertension • Arterial hypotension	• Proximal intracranial artery occlusion (i.e., MCA and ICA) • Symptomatic intracranial atherosclerotic disease
Hyperthermia	Transcranial Doppler
Diabetes mellitus • Hyperglycemia	• Persisting arterial occlusion • Arterial reocclusion • Arterial blood flow steal
Sleep apnea (AHI ≥10 events/h)	Invasive angiography
	• Collateral failure

NIHSS, National Institutes of Health stroke scale; AHI, apnea/hypopnea index; MCA, middle cerebral artery; CTP, computer-to-plate (imaging); DWI, diffusion-weighted imaging; PWI, perfusion-weighted imaging; ICA, internal carotid artery.

Pathogenic link between sleep apnea and acute stroke deterioration

General pathogenic mechanisms

Immediate consequences of recurrent apnea episodes comprise hypoxemia, hypercapnia, overactivation of the autonomic nervous system, and intrathoracic pressure changes [28]. The latter might lead to an increased risk of paradoxical embolism as OSA has been linked to the presence of a patent foramen ovale [29]. Apnea-induced autonomic effects can result in both elevated blood pressure and cardiac arrhythmias (e.g., sinus arrest and atrioventricular block), accompanied by reductions in blood pressure [28,30]. An efficient cerebral autoregulatory response to systemic hemodynamic oscillations is crucial to compensate for acute and chronic changes in cerebral perfusion pressure and to avoid critical hypo- or hyperperfusion of the brain tissue. However, in patients with ischemic stroke, hemodynamically compromised tissue is supplied by maximally or nearly maximally dilated arterioles and vasomotor reserve may become exhausted [31]. Because cerebral perfusion abnormalities seem to play an important and perhaps critical role in acute stroke deterioration [12], multiple systemic factors such as repetitive changes in the blood pressure, cardiac output, and arterial blood gases may do harm by inducing further hypoperfusion through the ischemic penumbra vasculature with compromised vasomotor reserve. However, the direct effect of apnea-associated changes in systemic hemodynamics to the CBF at the time of neurological deterioration has not been demonstrated yet.

One transcranial Doppler (TCD) study found severely impaired cerebral vasoreactivity and increased arterial stiffness in patients with PSG-confirmed severe OSA, especially during apnea episodes [32]. Another study suggested that cerebral vasoreactivity may be impaired not only before or during episodes of apnea or hypopnea but also in general, even during wakefulness [33]. These cerebral vasoreactivity disturbances, which are most likely the consequence of an endothelial dysfunction (particularly of nitric oxide synthase and endo-thelin pathways) [34,35], seem to correlate in magnitude with the severity of sleep apnea quantified by the AHI. The fact that an impaired cerebral autoregulation may be a round-the-clock mechanism accompanied by a diminished vasomotor reserve supports our recent findings that patients with an acute ischemic stroke and arterial blood flow steal were more likely to have a higher risk of recurrent strokes [36].

Arterial blood flow steal

Cerebral vasomotor reactivity is closely interrelated to the arterial level of CO_2 and CBF changes have been documented using TCD during episodes of voluntary breath-holding or inhalation of CO_2 [31,37]. Under ischemic conditions, the affected vessels are less responsive to vasodilatory stimuli like CO_2 as they are already maximally or nearly maximally dilated to compensate for an arterial occlusion or are affected by acidosis [38]. Their vasomotor capacity is also decreased if compared to nonaffected vessels that dilate more and change pressure gradients unfavorably for the ischemic tissues. Thus, blood flow diversion into nonaffected brain tissue (along the path of least resistance) is expected to occur and may facilitate further hypoperfusion through the ischemic penumbra. Intracranial arterial blood flow steal can be noninvasively detected in real-time and quantified by TCD as mean flow velocity reduction during spontaneous or voluntary breath-holding [39]. This has been described as the hemodynamic steal mechanism that can lead to clinical deterioration, termed reversed Robin Hood syndrome (RRHS):

$$Steal\ magnitude\ (\%) = \frac{MFV_{min} - MFV_{baseline}}{MFV_{baseline}} \times 100$$

where MFV_{min} is the minimal mean flow velocity detected at the time of vasodilation and velocity increase in the unaffected vessels. Note that this usually occurs 15–25 s from the beginning of voluntary breath-holding. Using TCD, the steal is detectable at the level of the circle of Willis, but a similar mechanism may exist at arteries beyond the first- and second-level branching.

Clinical evidence of the arterial blood flow steal

Our group has recently shown that the presence of an intracranial blood flow steal in ischemic stroke patients with an acute proximal arterial occlusion and excessive daytime sleepiness may be related to greater neurological deterioration during hospitalization [39]. More specifically, consecutive patients with acute cerebral ischemia admitted within 48 hours from symptom onset underwent serial NIHSS score examinations and bilateral TCD monitoring with voluntary breath-holding. Arterial steal was defined as an MFV decrease in the affected vessel at the time of presumed hypercapnia-induced velocity increase in the normal (nonaffected) vessel. The steal magnitude (SM, %) was quantified as the maximum negative percent velocity reduction during breath-holding. Arterial blood flow steal was considered present when SM was negative, that is, SM <0 in the affected vessel. Neurological deterioration was defined as an increase of ≥2 points in the NIHSS score within 48 hours from symptom onset. Patients with other known causes of clinical or neurological deterioration, including arterial reocclusion, continuing embolization, edema with mass effect, cardiovascular instability, and hemorrhagic transformation were excluded from the study. Daytime sleepiness preceding stroke was assessed by the Epworth sleepiness scale (ESS) and was considered abnormal when the score was >10 points. The likelihood of having sleep apnea was assessed by the Berlin questionnaire.

Among 153 studied patients, 21 (14%) had arterial blood flow steal with an average SM of –20%. In 11 (7%) patients, this steal was accompanied by a neurological deterioration. Reversed Robin Hood syndrome was most common in patients with proximal arterial occlusions (17% vs. 1%; P< 0.001) and in those with both arterial occlusions and excessive daytime sleepiness (40% vs. 5%; P=0.003). Excessive daytime sleepiness appeared to be significantly associated with RRHS. The likelihood of sleep apnea (assessed by the Berlin questionnaire) did not appear as a factor independently associated with the steal; however, the majority of patients with excessive daytime sleepiness had Berlin scores predictive of sleep apnea.

These data highlight the need to pay more attention to patients with persisting arterial occlusions and excessive daytime sleepiness as these two conditions may lead to hemodynamic compromise and subsequent clinical deterioration. Patients with symptomatic arterial blood flow steal had a greater need for collateral flow recruitment, because the underlying pathogenic mechanism of cerebral ischemia in the vast majority of studied patients with RRHS was large-artery atherothrombotic stroke (91%) [39]. Interestingly, collateral failure in persisting arterial occlusion appears to be one of the most relevant pathogenic mechanisms and independent predictors for acute stroke deterioration [40]. Thus, we hypothesized that these collaterals appeared insufficient to fully compensate during sleep and transient hypercapnia.

The main limitations of this study were the lack of blood gas measurements and overnight sleep studies leaving any causal relationship between respiratory function and neurological deterioration, thus far, speculative.

Future directions

Noninvasive ventilatory correction for acute ischemic stroke

In acute ischemic stroke patients, ischemic penumbra may be present for many hours and amenable to reversal. Consequently, any treatment that potentially augments cerebral perfusion may be justified [41]. Administration of oxygen, as is commonly performed in many stroke units, may not be sufficient to reverse the intracranial steal that may result in acute deterioration in stroke patients with sleep apnea. Treatment options for sleep apnea include postural changes and noninvasive ventilatory correction, with either continuous positive airway pressure (CPAP) or bi-level positive airway pressure (BiPAP). Although several studies have been conducted to demonstrate the safety and the beneficial effects of CPAP and BiPAP on improved quality of life and reduced cardio- and cerebrovascular morbidity and mortality in the general population [42,43], their role in acute ischemic stroke patients remains to be elucidated. To date, most recent stroke guidelines are silent in terms of recommendations for management of sleep-disordered breathing during hospitalization of acute stroke patients, not to mention the acute phase of stroke [44]. At least 10 studies investigated the effects of mechanical ventilation in stroke patients, whereas in most of these studies, treatment was initiated beyond the (hyper-) acute phase of stroke and aimed at safety and feasibility rather than an acute effect [45–48].

A recent study, investigating safety and tolerability of BiPAP treatment initiated within the first 24 hours of admission to the hospital, pointed to a potential short-term effect of this treatment [49]. Acute ischemic stroke patients with proximal arterial occlusions and excessive sleepiness or known OSA showed a trend toward better neurological recovery during the hospital course than those who did not receive noninvasive ventilatory correction (P=0.078). Another study assessed the feasibility of CPAP treatment initiated in the first night after stroke [50]. Overall, 50 patients were randomly assigned to the CPAP therapy group or to a control group and underwent PSG on the fourth night. Treated patients received CPAP therapy for three nights, starting the first night after stroke onset and for an additional four nights, when PSG revealed an AHI of >10 events/hour. The primary end point was feasibility defined as AHI reduction under CPAP treatment, nursing workload, and CPAP adherence. The investigators found that CPAP therapy initiated in the first night after stroke seems to be feasible as well as safe, and there was a trend toward greater NIHSS score improvement until day eight in the patients on CPAP (2.00 vs. 1.40, P=0.092), and a significantly greater NIHSS score improvement in patients with excellent CPAP use when compared with control patients (2.30 vs. 1.40, P=0.022).

However, further research is needed to determine in a prospective and randomized fashion whether noninvasive ventilatory correction can reduce the risk of acute stroke deterioration, improve functional outcomes, and decrease early mortality in acute ischemic stroke patients with or without sleep apnea. Novel methods of mechanical ventilation, such as auto-titrating ventilation devices that search pressures and adapt pressure settings from breath to breath, may be considered. Acute ischemic stroke and transient ischemic attack (TIA) patients have shown good tolerability to these promising devices [51,52].

Management of acute stroke patients with sleep apnea

Although sleep apnea is increasingly recognized by the stroke community as a serious disorder that contributes to worse outcomes and increased mortality in acute ischemic stroke patients, too little has been done yet to implement appropriate guidance and support into national stroke guidelines to break the proposed vicious cycle of transient hypoventilation–hypercapnia–hypoperfusion in these patients [53,54]. Expert opinion advocates that the suspicion of sleep apnea should trigger a comprehensive sleep evaluation, including sleep-oriented history and objective sleep testing by means of in-laboratory PSG or at least portable monitoring (so-called respiratory polygraphy) [54]. This approach may be reasonable in the ambulatory setting, but in the hospital setting, only a few stroke centers have access to sleep medicine for inpatient populations and even this access may not be continuously available. It is of particular interest to determine whether confirmation of sleep apnea with a complete overnight sleep study is necessary to initiate ventilatory correction, or whether treatment can be initiated based on clinical criteria alone. As follows, we describe specific steps taken in our institution:

1. Identify stroke patients who are admitted within 48 hours from symptom-onset. If neurological symptoms are fluctuating or progressing, consider brain perfusion augmentation.
2. Check if the occlusion location matches the size of an ischemic lesion on diffusion-weighted MRI and the neurological severity. If a mismatch is identified, potentially salvageable tissue may exist regardless of whether neurological fluctuation is present.
3. If a patient meets criteria 1 or 2, a comprehensive sleep history should be taken, and if available, an interview should include bed partner and family members.
4. Evaluate the patient clinically for:

   – excessive sleepiness
   – repetitive oxygen desaturations,
   – breathing pauses or shallow breathing and gasping/choking episodes while asleep.

5. We perform bilateral TCD arterial blood flow steal monitoring using diagnostic criteria as described in the previous sections. Briefly, two 2-MHz transducers fitted on a head-frame are placed on the temporal bone windows used to obtain a bilateral continuous measurement of the MFV in the middle cerebral arteries. The depths of insonation should be 50–65 mm bilaterally (alternatively, depth of occlusion location or worst residual flow) with a sample volume of 10 mm. Cerebrovascular reactivity is measured by means of a breath-holding index examination [37] or spontaneously if an uncooperative patient falls asleep. Arterial blood flow steal is defined as any MFV decrease in the affected vessel at the time of spontaneous or breath-holding induced velocity increase in the nonaffected vessel. The steal phenomenon is considered present when SM <0 in the affected vessel. After steal is documented on TCD, RRHS is diagnosed if recurrent neurological worsening by ≥2 points on NIHSS is documented without any other cause of neurological deterioration (Figure 9.1).

   Alternatively, patients may undergo a one-hour noninvasive sleep study preferably during the first night after admission. With a respiratory polygraphy device, nasal airflow, respiratory movements, and capillary oxygen saturation are monitored.
6. Patients with abnormal TCD or polygraphy findings receive bi-level positive airway pressure (settings of 10/5 cm water pressure) if sleep apnea or hypoventilation were previously not established. If sleep apnea was diagnosed previously, we ask relatives to bring the CPAP and BiPAP machines in use or provide the most recent pressure values from a sleep study done prior to the index stroke.

Conclusions

In summary, sleep apnea is associated with an increased risk of acute stroke deterioration within the first 72 hours after symptom onset. The pathogenic link between sleep apnea and acute deterioration in ischemic stroke patients is now a subject of clinical investigation. Because cerebral perfusion abnormalities seem to play an important, and perhaps critical role in acute stroke deterioration, multiple systemic factors such as repetitive changes in blood pressure, thoracic pressure, and cardiac output may do harm by inducing further hypoperfusion through the ischemic penumbra vasculature, where the vasomotor reserve may be even more compromised. Intracranial blood flow steal in response to changing and arterial blood gases like carbon dioxide play a pivotal role in clinical deterioration with RRHS.

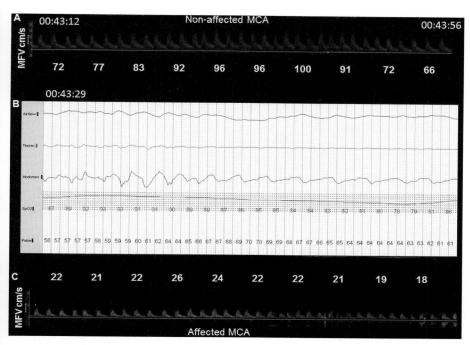

Figure 9.1. Case illustration: a 67-year-old woman admitted with a left-sided acute ischemic stroke had a baseline National Institutes of Health stroke scale score of 13 points. Initial transcranial Doppler (TCD) demonstrated a dampened flow of the left middle cerebral artery (MCA) (TIBI flow grade 3) at a depth of 42mm, indicating an acute M2-MCA occlusion. A comprehensive sleep history obtained shortly after admission revealed symptoms highly suggestive of sleep apnea with an Epworth sleepiness scale of 15 points (indicating excessive daytime sleepiness) and a Berlin questionnaire classifying her as high-risk for having sleep apnea. In the first night after admission, the patient was monitored simultaneously with both bilateral TCD (A, C) and respiratory polygraphy (B) for one hour while asleep. The illustration of the respiratory polygram shows an excerpt of a 30-s epoch of hypopnea/apnea (with an obstructive pattern) accompanied by an oxygen desaturation nadir of 78%. Simultaneously, mean flow velocity (MFV) increases in the nonaffected MCA (at 59mm) while MFV in the affected MCA (at 42mm) remains at first unchanged ("frozen") and subsequently drops, indicating exhausted vasomotor reactivity and arterial blood flow steal, respectively (Doppler spectra and the respiratory polygram are arranged in an offset manner). Steal magnitude (SM) was calculated using the highest and lowest MFV in the affected side during this apnea/hypopnea epoch. (SM = (21 cm/s − 26 cm/s − 26 cm/s) x 100 = −15%.)

Transcranial Doppler sonography provides a noninvasive and inexpensive vascular test that can be used to provide real-time physiological information in patients with suspected arterial blood flow steal. Noninvasive ventilatory correction in selected acute stroke patients could have a beneficial effect on sleep apnea and brain perfusion. This is a novel therapeutic target and the missing link in the pathogenesis of acute stroke deterioration in some patients. The hypothesis should be tested in a clinical trial.

References

1. Kwan J, Hand P. Early neurological deterioration in acute stroke: clinical characteristics and impact on outcome. *QJM* 2006; **99**: 625–33.

2. Weimar C, Mieck T, Buchthal J, et al. Neurologic worsening during the acute phase of ischemic stroke. *Arch Neurol* 2005; **62**: 393–7.

3. Audebert HJ, Pellkofer TS, Wimmer ML, et al. Progression in lacunar stroke is related to elevated acute phase parameters. *Eur Neurol* 2004; **51**: 125–31.
4. Saqqur M, Molina CA, Salam A, et al. Clinical deterioration after intravenous recombinant tissue plasminogen activator treatment: a multicenter transcranial Doppler study. *Stroke* 2007; **38**: 69–74.
5. Yamamoto H, Bogousslavsky J, van Melle G. Different predictors of neurological worsening in different causes of stroke. *Arch Neurol* 1998; **55**: 481–6.
6. Davalos A, Toni D, Iweins F, et al. Neurological deterioration in acute ischemic stroke: potential predictors and associated factors in the European Cooperative Acute Stroke Study (ECASS) I. *Stroke* 1999; **30**: 2631–6.
7. Tei H, Uchiyama S, Ohara K, et al. Deteriorating ischemic stroke in 4 clinical categories classified by the Oxfordshire Community Stroke Project. *Stroke* 2000; **31**: 2049–54.
8. Mohr JP, Caplan LR, Melski JW, et al. The Harvard Cooperative Stroke Registry: a prospective registry. *Neurology* 1978; **28**: 754–62.
9. Martí-Vilalta JL, Arboix A. The Barcelona Stroke Registry. *Eur Neurol* 1999; **41**: 135–42.
10. Park TS, Choi BJ, Lee TH, et al. Urgent recanalization with stenting for severe intracranial atherosclerosis after transient ischemic attack or minor stroke. *J Korean Neurosurg Soc* 2011; **50**: 322–6.
11. Barlinn K, Kepplinger J, Kolieskova S, et al. Symptomatic intracranial atherosclerotic disease in acute cerebral ischemia: frequency, clinical course and short-term outcome in a tertiary care hospital in the southeastern United States. *Stroke* 2012; **43**: A121.
12. Alawneh JA, Moustafa RR, Baron JC. Hemodynamic factors and perfusion abnormalities in early neurological deterioration. *Stroke* 2009; **40**: e443–50.
13. Ois A, Martinez-Rodriguez JE, Munteis E, et al. Steno-occlusive arterial disease and early neurological deterioration in acute ischemic stroke. *Cerebrovasc Dis* 2008; **25**: 151–6.
14. Rajajee V, Kidwell C, Starkman S, et al. Early MRI and outcomes of untreated patients with mild or improving ischemic stroke. *Neurology* 2006; **67**: 980–4.
15. Toni D, Fiorelli M, Gentile M, et al. Progressing neurological deficit secondary to acute ischemic stroke. A study on predictability, pathogenesis, and prognosis. *Arch Neurol* 1995; **52**: 670–5.
16. Alexandrov AV, Grotta JC. Arterial reocclusion in stroke patients treated with intravenous tissue plasminogen. *Neurology* 2002; **59**: 862–7.
17. Janjua N, Alkawi A, Suri MF, et al. Impact of arterial reocclusion and distal fragmentation during thrombolysis among patients with acute ischemic stroke. *AJNR Am J Neuroradiol* 2008; **29**: 253–8.
18. Rubiera M, Alvarez-Sabı́ ́n J, Ribo M, et al. Predictors of early arterial reocclusion after tissue plasminogen activator-induced recanalization in acute ischemic stroke. *Stroke* 2005; **36**: 1452–6.
19. Valton L, Larrue V, le Traon AP, et al. Microembolic signals and risk of early recurrence in patients with stroke or transient ischemic attack. *Stroke* 1998; **29**: 2125–8.
20. Davalos A, Castillo J, Pumar JM, et al. Body temperature and fibrinogen are related to early neurological deterioration in acute ischemic stroke. *Cerebrovasc Dis* 1997; **7**: 64–9.
21. Parsons MW, Barber PA, Desmond PM, et al. Acute hyperglycemia adversely affects stroke outcome: a magnetic resonance imaging and spectroscopy study. *Ann Neurol* 2002; **52**: 20–8.
22. Toni D, Fiorelli M, Zanette EM, et al. Early spontaneous improvement and deterioration of ischemic stroke patients. A serial study with transcranial Doppler ultrasonography. *Stroke* 1998; **29**: 1144–8.
23. Alvarez FJ, Segura T, Castellanos M, et al. Cerebral hemodynamic reserve and early neurologic deterioration in acute ischemic stroke. *J Cereb Blood Flow Metab* 2004; **24**: 1267–71.
24. Iranzo A, Santamaría J, Berenguer J, et al. Prevalence and clinical importance of sleep apnea in the first night after cerebral infarction. *Neurology* 2002; **58**: 911–16.
25. Arzt M, Young T, Finn L, et al. Association of sleep disordered breathing and the

occurrence of stroke. *Am J Respir Crit Care Med* 2005; **172**: 1447–51.

26. Yaggi HK, Concato J, Kernan WN, et al. Obstructive sleep apnea as a risk factor for stroke and death. *N Engl J Med* 2005; **353**: 2034–41.

27. Bassetti CL, Milanova M, Gugger M. Sleep-disordered breathing and acute ischemic stroke: diagnosis, risk factors, treatment, evolution, and long-term clinical outcome. *Stroke* 2006; **37**: 967–72.

28. Shamsuzzaman AS, Gersh BJ, Somers VK. Obstructive sleep apnea: implications for cardiac and vascular disease. *JAMA* 2003; **290**: 1906–14.

29. Lau EM, Yee BJ, Grunstein RR, et al. Patent foramen ovale and obstructive sleep apnea: a new association? *Sleep Med Rev* 2010; **14**: 391–5.

30. Wolk R, Kara T, Somers VK. Sleep-disordered breathing and cardiovascular disease. *Circulation* 2003; **108**: 9–12.

31. Ringelstein EB, Sievers C, Ecker S, et al. Noninvasive assessment of CO2-induced cerebral vasomotor response in normal individuals and patients with internal carotid artery occlusions. *Stroke* 1988; **19**: 963–9.

32. Furtner M, Staudacher M, Frauscher B, et al. Cerebral vasoreactivity decreases overnight in severe obstructive sleep apnea syndrome: a study of cerebral hemodynamics. *Sleep Med* 2009; **10**: 875–81.

33. Nasr N, Pavy-Le Traon A, Czosnyka M, et al. Cerebral autoregulation in patients with obstructive sleep apnea syndrome during wakefulness. *Eur J Neurol* 2009; **16**: 386–91.

34. Ip MS, Lam B, Chan LY, et al. Circulating nitric oxide is suppressed in obstructive sleep apnea and is reversed by nasal continuous airway pressure. *Am J Respir Crit Care Med* 2000; **162**: 2166–71.

35. Phillips RA, Narkiewicz K, Pesek CA, et al. Effects of obstructive sleep apnea on endothelin-1 and blood pressure. *J Hypertens* 1999; **17**: 61–6.

36. Palazzo P, Balucani C, Barlinn K, et al. Association of reversed Robin Hood syndrome with risk of stroke recurrence. *Neurology* 2010; **75**: 2003–8.

37. Markus HS, Harrison MJ. Estimation of cerebrovascular reactivity using transcranial Doppler, including the use of breath-holding as the vasodilatory stimulus. *Stroke* 1992; **23**: 668–73.

38. Silvestrini M, Vernieri F, Pasqualetti P, et al. Impaired cerebral vasoreactivity and risk of stroke in patients with asymptomatic carotid artery stenosis. *JAMA* 2000; **283**: 2122–7.

39. Alexandrov AV, Nguyen HT, Rubiera M, et al. Prevalence and risk factors associated with reversed Robin Hood syndrome in acute ischemic stroke. *Stroke* 2009; **40**: 2738–42.

40. Ali LK, Saver JL. The ischemic stroke patient who worsens: new assessment and management approaches. *Rev Neurol Dis* 2007; **4**: 85–91.

41. Fisher M, Garcia JH. Evolving stroke and the ischemic penumbra. *Neurology.* 1996; **47**: 884–8.

42. Ballester E, Badia JR, Hernandez L, et al. Evidence of the effectiveness of continuous positive airway pressure in the treatment of sleep apnea/hypopnea syndrome. *Am J Respir Crit Care Med* 1999; **159**: 495–501.

43. Jenkinson C, Davies RJ, Mullins R, et al. Comparison of therapeutic and subtherapeutic nasal continuous positive airway pressure for obstructive sleep apnoea: a randomised prospective parallel trial. *Lancet* 1999; **353**: 2100–5.

44. Adams HP Jr, del Zoppo G, Alberts MJ, et al. Guidelines for the early management of adults with ischemic stroke: a guideline from the American Heart Association/ American Stroke Association Stroke Council, Clinical Cardiology Council, Cardiovascular Radiology and Intervention Council, and the Atherosclerotic Peripheral Vascular Disease and Quality of Care Outcomes in Research Interdisciplinary Working Groups: the American Academy of Neurology affirms the value of this guideline as an educational tool for neurologists. *Circulation* 2007; **115**: e478–534.

45. Parra O, Sánchez-Armengol A, Bonnin M, et al. Early treatment of obstructive apnoea and stroke outcome: a randomised controlled trial. *Eur Respir J* 2011; **37**: 1128–36.

46. Ryan CM, Bayley M, Green R, et al. Influence of continuous positive airway

pressure on outcomes of rehabilitation in stroke patients with obstructive sleep apnea. *Stroke* 2011; **42**: 1062–7.

47. Martinez-Garcia MA, Soler-Cataluna JJ, Ejarque-Martinez L, et al. Continuous positive airway pressure treatment reduces mortality in patients with ischemic stroke and obstructive sleep apnea, a 5-year follow-up study. *Am J Respir Crit Care Med* 2009; **180**: 36–41.

48. Hermann DM, Bassetti CL. Sleep-related breathing and sleep-wake disturbances in ischemic stroke. *Neurology* 2009; **73**: 1313–22.

49. Tsivgoulis G, Zhang Y, Alexandrov AW, et al. Safety and tolerability of early noninvasive ventilatory correction using bilevel positive airway pressure in acute ischemic stroke. *Stroke* 2011; **42**: 1030–4.

50. Minnerup J, Ritter MA, Wersching H, et al. Continuous positive airway pressure ventilation for acute ischemic stroke: a randomized feasibility study. *Stroke* 2012; **43**: 1137–9.

51. Bravata DM, Concato J, Fried T, et al. Auto-titrating continuous positive airway pressure for patients with acute transient ischemic attack: a randomized feasibility trial. *Stroke* 2010; **41**: 1464–70.

52. Scala R, Turkington PM, Wanklyn P, et al. Acceptance, effectiveness and safety of continuous positive airway pressure in acute stroke: a pilot study. *Respir Med* 2009; **103**: 59–66.

53. Sharma VK, Teoh HL, Paliwal PR, et al. Reversed Robin Hood syndrome in a patient with luxury perfusion after acute ischemic stroke. *Circulation*. 2011; **123**: e243–4.

54. Epstein LJ, Kristo D, Strollo PJ Jr, et al. Clinical guideline for the evaluation, management and long-term care of obstructive sleep apnea in adults. *J Clin Sleep Med* 2009; **5**: 263–76.

Chapter 1

Effect of continuous positive airway pressure on stroke risk factors and stroke

Malcolm Kohler and John R. Stradling

Continuous positive airway pressure

Obstructive sleep apnea (OSA) is characterized by a repetitive collapse of the pharynx during sleep resulting in apnea and hypopnea, which are associated with intrathoracic pressure changes, oxygen desaturations, and arousals from sleep. It was not until 1982, when Colin Sullivan in Australia invented continuous nasal positive airway pressure ventilation (CPAP), that a fully effective, noninvasive treatment for OSA became available [1]. Nocturnal application of CPAP via a nasal or face mask is the standard therapy for patients with obstructive sleep apnea syndrome (OSAS). The positive airflow pressure that is generated by an airflow turbine pump forces open the pharynx, thereby preventing apneas, hypopneas, snoring, and any acute physiological consequences of OSA. Continuous positive airway pressure has been shown to improve daytime symptoms such as excessive sleepiness, quality of life, blood pressure, and other measures of cardiovascular risk in patients with moderate to severe OSAS [2,3]. There is also some evidence that CPAP has the same beneficial effects on sleepiness and quality of life in patients with minimally symptomatic OSA without excessive daytime sleepiness [2]. As OSAS is often a lifelong condition, CPAP usually needs to be used indefinitely. Approximately 30%–50% of all patients diagnosed with OSAS will not tolerate CPAP in the long term, and nightly adherence to this therapy shows a considerable interindividual variability, which is particularly true for patients with milder forms of OSA who may not perceive improvement in daytime symptoms such as sleepiness with this treatment [4,5]. However, currently there is no data on the minimum time of CPAP use per night that is required for patients to fully benefit from this therapy in terms of improvement in symptoms, quality of life, blood pressure, or any other measure of cardiovascular risk. This needs to be taken into account when considering the effects of CPAP on postulated stroke risk factors and cerebrovascular events, which are discussed in the following sections of this chapter.

Effects of continuous positive airway pressure on stroke risk factors

In the following section, the impact of CPAP therapy on major treatable risk factors for cerebrovascular atherosclerotic disease including arterial hypertension, diabetes mellitus, and dyslipidemia will be reviewed. As atrial fibrillation (AF) is recognized as an

---

Sleep, Stroke, and Cardiovascular Disease, ed. Antonio Culebras. Published by Cambridge University Press. © Cambridge University Press 2013.

important risk factor for thromboembolic cerebrovascular disease, this chapter also includes a discussion on the effect of CPAP treatment on AF.

Effect of continuous positive airway pressure on blood pressure

The repetitive episodes of obstructive apneas are often associated with arousals and intermittent hypoxia, both of which lead to increased sympathetic nervous system activity and consequent marked transient increases in arterial blood pressure of up to 60–80 mmHg (Figure 10.1). The activation of the sympathetic nervous system is also associated with an augmented production of catecholamines (e.g., norepinephrine) during the night, which are released into the circulation and may thereby contribute to the development of sustained hypertension [6,7]. The nocturnal sympathetic nervous system activation and consequently higher sleep-related blood pressure may attenuate or abolish the physiological nocturnal dipping of blood pressure [3,8]. Augmented sympathetic activation may also increase arterial stiffness, impair endothelial function, and blunt baroreflex sensitivity, all of which have been shown to contribute to the development of arterial hypertension [8, 9]. In population-based prospective cohort studies, OSAS has repeatedly been associated with an increased risk for the development of arterial hypertension [10].

Continuous positive airway pressure treatment has been shown to not only effectively abolish apnea, hypopnoea, and oxygen desaturations, but also decrease arousal frequency and thus suppress acute blood pressure swings (Figure 10.2). Based on the acute physiological effects of CPAP on nocturnal blood pressure swings, and the promising findings of numerous uncontrolled studies, several randomized controlled trials looking at the effect of CPAP on 24-hour ambulatory blood pressure have been conducted in recent years. The results of these randomized controlled trials have established that CPAP treatment of symptomatic patients with moderate to severe OSAS lowers blood pressure to some extent [3,6,8,11–14]. Most of these studies reported a reduction in blood pressure between 2 and 10 mmHg after several weeks of CPAP therapy [8, 13]. However, although it is generally accepted that CPAP has a beneficial effect on arterial hypertension in patients with OSAS,

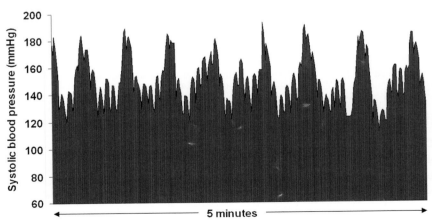

Figure 10.1. Nocturnal systolic blood pressure over five minutes in a patient with obstructive sleep apnea is shown (beat-to-beat blood pressure measured with a Finapres® device). Multiple arousal-related rises in blood pressure up to 60 mmHg, which correspond to the end of the apneas, can be noted.

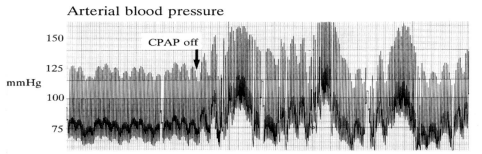

Figure 10.2. The effect of continuous positive airway pressure (CPAP) on blood pressure swings is illustrated.When the CPAP device is switched off, arousal-related blood pressure surges return immediately.

there is still a debate about the underlying mechanisms of this favorable effect. In a large randomized controlled trial on the impact of four weeks of CPAP therapy on various measures of cardiovascular risk, which included 102 middle-aged males with moderate to severe OSAS, the reduction in 24-hour ambulatory blood pressure was accompanied by a reduction in 24-hour urine catecholamine excretion and arterial stiffness as well as by an improvement in baroreflex sensitivity, a measure of sympathovagal balance [8]. In the same trial, CPAP treatment had no effect on measures of systemic inflammation such as highly sensitive C-reactive protein (hsCRP) [7]. Thus the findings of the latter study suggest that CPAP reduces blood pressure primarily through an improvement in sympathovagal balance. In addition, there is evidence from randomized controlled trials that CPAP therapy in OSA also improves oxidative stress and endothelial dysfunction, both recognized as important factors contributing to the development of arterial hypertension [9,15].

The effect of CPAP on systemic blood pressure in patients with OSAS seems to depend on the severity of sleep-disordered breathing, daytime sleepiness, extent of obesity, and the hours of nightly CPAP use [3,14,16]. In the randomized, sham-controlled trial by Pepperell and colleagues [3], which included 118 male OSAS patients, the reduction in mean ambulatory 24-hour blood pressure with CPAP was only 1.1 mmHg in patients with an oxygen desaturation index (ODI) below the median of the studied population (ODI <33/hour), whereas it was 5.1 mmHg in patients with an ODI above the median (ODI >33/hour). In the meta-analysis by Haentjens et al. [14], a meta-regression that included 572 individuals (12 trials) estimated the 24-hour ambulatory mean blood pressure to decrease by 0.89 mmHg per 10-point increase in the AHI at study entry (see following discussion). However, the findings of an uncontrolled study on predictors of blood pressure fall with CPAP treatment of OSAS by Robinson et al. [16]suggest that daytime sleepiness and body mass index (BMI), but not the sleep-study severity of sleep-disordered breathing, are independently associated with the fall in blood pressure after six months of CPAP therapy. Recent findings suggest that the beneficial effects of CPAP on blood pressure are mainly found in those patients who show a favorable adherence to treatment (e.g., more than four hours per night) [14,17]. However, more evidence from well-designed studies is needed to clarify questions such as the predictors of likely benefit and the minimum hours of CPAP therapy necessary to achieve a full beneficial effect on blood pressure, in a typical population of patients with OSA.

Interestingly, there is less evidence from randomized controlled trials that CPAP significantly lowers office blood pressure [8]. This is likely to be due to difficulties in detecting small changes in blood pressure with the less accurate and reproducible office measurements ascribed to variable "white coat" effects [18]. However, the results of a recently published randomized controlled trial suggest that effects of CPAP on domiciliary blood pressure are most pronounced in the morning, possibly due to a reduction in the augmented sympathetic activity during the night [9]. This needs to be taken into account when treatment effects of CPAP on blood pressure are evaluated in routine clinical practice.

To date, four meta-analyses have been published on the impact of CPAP therapy on blood pressure [6,11,14,19]. The meta-analysis by Haentjens et al. [14]. included 572 patients from 12 randomized controlled studies in which ambulatory 24-hour blood pressure was measured. Haentjens and colleagues [14]found a modest average reduction of the mean blood pressure of 1.9 mmHg with CPAP therapy, which is comparable to the findings of McDaid et al. [19](–2.1 mmHg). The meta-analyses by Bazzano et al. [6] and Alajmi et al. [11] were restricted to randomized controlled trials with a treatment duration of at least two weeks. The average reduction in mean blood pressure with CPAP compared to controls was -2.2 mmHg in the meta-analysis by Bazzano et al. [6] and –1.5 mmHg in the one by Alajmi et al. [11].The small effects of CPAP treatment on blood pressure found in these meta-analyses may be related to methodological differences among the trials, including different study populations, such as sleepy patients versus minimally symptomatic or non-sleepy patients, the proportion of patients with hypertension or on antihypertensive medication included, different sample sizes, different techniques used for blood pressure measurements (e.g., single time point versus 24-hour blood pressure versus beat-to-beat blood pressure measurements), and differences in the duration of the intervention time. However, the largest reduction in mean blood pressure (9.9 mmHg) was observed in a study in which the duration of the CPAP treatment intervention was nine weeks, and beat-to-beat blood pressure was measured in hospital over 19 hours with limited mobility, a technique with a higher reproducibility than conventional intermittent methods of blood pressure measurement [13].

Effect of continuous positive airway pressure on blood pressure in minimally symptomatic or non-sleepy obstructive sleep apnea patients

The prevalence of asymptomatic or minimally symptomatic OSA has been reported to be as high as 30% in adult populations, making OSA one of the most common disorders of epidemiological interest [20]. Whether these minimally symptomatic OSA patients are also at increased risk of developing arterial hypertension is currently a matter of debate. In contrast to the fall in blood pressure seen in sleepy patients, Robinson et al. [21] found no significant fall in mean blood pressure with CPAP therapy in a randomized controlled trial including non-sleepy hypertensive patients with OSA. Similarly, Barbé and colleagues [22] found no significant effect of CPAP on blood pressure in a randomized controlled trial including 55 patients with OSA but no daytime sleepiness. However, a recently published Spanish multicenter controlled CPAP trial, including 359 hypertensive, non-sleepy OSA patients with an AHI of >19 events/h and an Epworth sleepiness score (ESS) of <11, has shown that one year of CPAP treatment reduces systolic and diastolic blood pressures

(−1.9 mmHg; 95% CI, −3.9 to +0.1 mmHg; and −2.2 mmHg, 95% CI, −3.5 to −0.9 mmHg, respectively) [17]. The most significant reduction in blood pressure was found in patients who used CPAP treatment for more than 5.6 hours per night, which perhaps implies two things: first, these individuals were more sleepy than was suggested by the ESS of <11 (hence their good CPAP compliance due to perceived benefits), and/or second, non-sleepy OSA patients need to be especially compliant with CPAP therapy in order to benefit from a clinically significant reduction in blood pressure [17].

Effect of continuous positive airway pressure on blood pressure in patients with obstructive sleep apnea and resistant hypertension

Obstructive sleep apnea syndrome has been proposed to be a risk factor for resistant hypertension, which is defined as repeatedly measured blood pressures ≥140/90 mmHg despite treatment with at least three antihypertensive drugs. Logan and colleagues [23] found that the prevalence of OSA (defined as an AHI of ≥10 events/h) in patients with resistant hypertension was 83%. Ruttanaumpawan et al. [24] reported a prevalence of OSA of 81% (defined as an AHI of ≥10 events/h) in patients with resistant hypertension compared to 55% in patients with controlled hypertension. More recently, OSA was suggested to be the most common secondary cause of hypertension associated with resistant hypertension [25]. The very high prevalence of OSA in these cross-sectional studies suggests that there may be a causal relationship between OSA and resistant hypertension.

In a randomized controlled trial looking at the effects of 3 months of CPAP therapy in patients with OSA and resistant hypertension, CPAP treatment was associated with a decrease in diastolic blood pressure of 5.0 mmHg [26]. Patients who used CPAP more than 5.8 hours per night showed an even greater reduction in daytime diastolic blood pressure (6.1 mmHg), 24-hour diastolic blood pressure (7.0 mmHg), and 24-hour systolic blood pressure (9.7 mmHg), emphasizing the importance of optimal CPAP adherence [26]. The results of this trial suggest that all patients with resistant hypertension should potentially be screened for OSA as CPAP therapy may lead to clinically significant reductions in blood pressure, greater than can be achieved with drugs alone.

Effect of continuous positive airway pressure on glucose metabolism

Obstructive sleep apnea and type 2 diabetes are both conditions that are closely associated with obesity, with a high prevalence of OSA in those patients with type 2 diabetes, and high levels of type 2 diabetes in patients with OSA [27]. However, the causative effect of each condition on the other, independent of obesity, is more difficult to determine and still a matter of debate. Based on the findings of observational cohort studies mentioned earlier, it can be hypothesized that CPAP treatment of patients with OSA would alleviate insulin resistance and improve glucose metabolism, perhaps through resolution of the intermittent hypoxia and arousal-associated sympathetic activation. The only method to establish a truly obesity-independent causal relationship between OSA and increased insulin resistance in humans is to perform a randomized controlled interventional trial investigating the effects of CPAP therapy on insulin resistance.

Randomized controlled trials on the effect of continuous positive airway pressure on insulin resistance

Results from four randomized controlled trials on the effect of CPAP treatment on glucose metabolism in patients with OSA have been published to date. West and colleagues [28] randomized 42 obese patients with type 2 diabetes and OSA to either three months of therapeutic or subtherapeutic CPAP, and evaluated the treatment effect on glucose metabolism and insulin sensitivity. The authors found no improvement in insulin sensitivity, or in other measures of glycemic control, after three months of therapeutic CPAP, when compared to subtherapeutic CPAP. The relatively low mean compliance with therapeutic and subtherapeutic CPAP (3.6 ± 2.8 and 3.3 ± 3.0 hours per night, respectively) in this trial raised the question whether the negative finding of the study can be explained by insufficient use of CPAP. However, the authors did not find a correlation between CPAP use and change in measures of glycemic control, suggesting that the finding cannot be explained solely by insufficient adherence to CPAP.

Another randomized controlled crossover trial from the U.K., which included 34 non-diabetic, mostly obese OSA patients, evaluated the effects of six weeks of CPAP on fasting blood glucose and insulin resistance. Six weeks of therapeutic CPAP had no statistically significant effect on fasting glucose and insulin resistance compared to subtherapeutic CPAP, again irrespective of the patients' compliance to treatment [29]. The authors of this trial hypothesized that there might be a threshold level of obesity where excess body fat is the principal determinant of insulin sensitivity irrespective of the presence of OSA or its severity, and thus CPAP treatment may not be expected to improve glucose metabolism in such patients.

More recently, a trial from China investigated the effects of one week of CPAP treatment on insulin sensitivity in 61 non-diabetic, overweight (mean BMI 27.5) Asian patients with OSA [30]. Insulin sensitivity, as assessed by the short insulin tolerance test (SITT), increased significantly in patients randomized to therapeutic CPAP, compared to patients who received subtherapeutic CPAP. Interestingly, insulin resistance, as assessed by the homeostatic model assessment (HOMA), did not improve significantly with therapeutic CPAP in the latter trial. This observed discrepancy may possibly be explained first by the fact that the two different techniques used to estimate insulin sensitivity probably represent different metabolic aspects of insulin resistance and, second, that this Chinese population was specifically non-diabetic. Interestingly, after 12 weeks of CPAP, no significant difference in insulin sensitivity remained when compared to baseline, except in a more obese subgroup; contrary to the hypothesis advanced previously.

In a randomized controlled trial by Kohler and colleagues [9], which included 41 obese patients with OSA, fourteen days of CPAP treatment withdrawal had no effect on glucose metabolism and insulin resistance. This was despite CPAP withdrawal being associated with a rapid recurrence of OSA leading to clear physiological effects on blood pressure and vascular function. A possible methodological explanation for this negative finding may be that insulin resistance was not the primary outcome of the study, and consequently this trial did not specifically include patients with abnormal glucose metabolism, thus resulting in only a small proportion of patients with diagnosed diabetes mellitus (approximately 20%).

The described randomized controlled trials have important differences regarding the selected patient populations (diabetic versus non-diabetic), the duration of the intervention period, and the methods used to assess insulin resistance and glucose metabolism. However, none of these trials found an improvement of insulin resistance assessed by HOMA. It can be argued that, in some of these trials, CPAP compliance was not sufficient to modify the changes in insulin resistance caused by OSA, or that in some patients, particularly in those with established diabetes, insulin resistance was too severe for significant modification by CPAP therapy, but overall the results argue against a clinically important positive effect of CPAP treatment on glucose metabolism. To answer the question whether OSA is causally related to insulin resistance and diabetes, and whether this should influence treatment decisions, requires more data from randomized controlled trials with more carefully defined patients.

Effect of continuous positive airway pressure on blood lipids

Given that patients with OSA are usually obese, it is not surprising that lipid abnormalities occur commonly. Hypercholesterolemia, although a risk factor for atherosclerosis, is only a weak risk factor for ischemic stroke [31]. Although statins reduce cholesterol and stroke risk, other cholesterol lowering strategies do not, implying that the effects of statins may be by alternative therapeutic pathways such as reduced prothrombotic tendency, reduced systemic inflammation, or improved endothelial function [32]. This means that a randomized controlled trial of CPAP indicating an effect on lipid metabolism would not necessarily imply a consequential altered stroke risk.

The parallel randomized controlled trial by Robinson et al. [33], including 213 patients with moderate to severe symptomatic OSA, measured cholesterol levels before and after a month of CPAP versus sham CPAP. In the group receiving therapeutic CPAP, there was a significant fall of cholesterol of 0.28 mmol/L. However, when compared to the control group, this only reached a significance level of P=0.06. In a crossover, sham-placebo controlled trial of CPAP in patients with OSA, the greater fall in cholesterol with CPAP was not significant, although the confidence intervals of the difference between the two arms only excluded a difference of >0.5 mmol/L [29]. More recently, a parallel randomized controlled trial of two months CPAP versus sham CPAP, in 29 patients (BMI <35) with severe OSA, looked at 24-hour cholesterol and triglyceride profiles based on seven blood samples taken across 24 hours. There was a significant effect on both triglycerides and cholesterol, with the treatment effect on cholesterol being 0.19 mmol/L [34]. This would likely reduce cardiac vascular events, but as discussed earlier, may not influence stroke rate.

A more recent alternative approach to study the short-term effects of sleep apnea on blood lipids has been to withdraw CPAP therapy from patients with OSA for a period of two weeks in comparison to a parallel group remaining on CPAP [9]. In this study, 41 highly CPAP compliant patients with OSA were included. There was no change in total cholesterol in the group experiencing a return of their OSA, but again, the power of the study was such that only a difference between groups of >0.4 mol/L was excluded. However, there was actually a small but statistically significant fall in triglycerides (0.2 mmol/L) in the group experiencing a return of their OSA.

Thus, it appears that more severe OSA is associated with a small rise in cholesterol with less evidence for a difference in fasting triglycerides. However, the effect of CPAP therapy on cholesterol seems to be very small and would be easily achieved through the use of statin therapy.

Effect of continuous positive airway pressure on atrial fibrillation

Atrial fibrillation is clearly a risk factor for stroke and may be provoked by OSA. How OSA might increase susceptibility to AF is not known. The increased sympathetic drive seen in patients with OSA may be important [18], particularly in association with the enhanced vagal tone that occurs during apneas [35], which would be expected to reduce the atrial effective refractory period [36]. However, recent evidence suggests that the considerable subatmospheric pressures generated in the thorax during obstructive apneas may distend vascular structures, including the atria, and may thereby alter the electrophysiology relevant to AF [37, 38].

Should OSA be associated with AF, then this would clearly be an important finding. Furthermore, if CPAP were shown to reduce the occurrence of AF (or reoccurrence following conversion therapy), then this would be of even greater significance. Many studies have found an association between OSA and AF with, for example, an approximate 25% greater risk of AF recurrence after catheter ablation in those with compared to those without OSA [39], but there have been no randomized controlled trials of CPAP on AF recurrence. Two nonrandomized studies have compared patients with OSA who use their CPAP, with those who do not or who were not prescribed it. Patel et al. [40] looked at 3000 patients having pulmonary vein isolation therapy for AF; 21% of the studied patients had OSA. After an average follow-up period of 32 months, 79% of the CPAP users did not experience AF recurrence, compared to 68% in the CPAP non-user group (P=0.003).

A smaller study by Kanagala et al. [41] included 39 OSA patients with AF/atrial flutter referred for DC cardioversion. Twenty-seven of the 39 patients either were not or were poorly treated with CPAP. Recurrence of AF one year after cardioversion was noted in 82% of these patients, whereas AF recurrence was only observed in 42% of patients well treated with CPAP (P=0.034). However, such nonrandomized studies using CPAP non-compliant OSA patients as controls remain essentially hypothesis-generating studies. Therefore, robust randomized controlled interventional trials in this area are urgently needed to establish a possible causal relationship between OSA and AF.

Effect of continuous positive airway pressure on stroke

Preliminary evidence from general and OSA population cohorts, showing that OSA precedes stroke and may therefore contribute to the development of stroke [42–44], and the high prevalence (>50%) of OSA observed in patients with stroke or TIA suggest that there may be a causal relationship between OSA and cerebrovascular events. Based on these observations and the positive effect of OSA treatment on some stroke risk factors, it is to be expected that treatment of OSA with CPAP might have a beneficial effect on the rate of first-time-ever stroke, TIA, or recurrent cerebrovascular events. It is still a matter of debate whether CPAP therapy has a positive impact on cerebrovascular event rates; this is because there are no published data from randomized controlled trials investigating the effects of CPAP on stroke/TIA incidence in OSA patients without a history of previous cerebrovascular events. In addition, there is very little data from randomized controlled studies on the effect of CPAP on stroke outcomes and recurrence rates of cerebrovascular events, possibly reflecting the difficulties of performing such rigorous trials in patients with acute cerebrovascular events. However, it has recently been shown by European- and U.S.-based research groups that such trials are feasible in patients with acute stroke or TIA [45–48]. There is some evidence supporting the hypothesis that early treatment of OSA in patients with acute stroke may have a protective effect on the brain; CPAP prevents recurrent hypoxemia, cerebral blood flow fluctuations, and blood pressure swings associated with obstructive apnea, all of which may further damage the area of the ischemic penumbra in the brain of stroke patients [49, 50].

The results of nonrandomized studies suggest that CPAP may improve mortality and prevent new vascular events after ischemic stroke in patients with OSA [51–53].

In the randomized controlled trial by Parra et al. [45], which assessed the impact of two years of CPAP treatment on functional outcome, quality of life, appearance of new cardiovascular events, and mortality in patients with acute ischemic stroke, 140 patients with an AHI of ≥20 events/h were included. Three to six days after stroke onset, 71 patients were randomized to CPAP and 69 patients to conventional treatment for two years. Continuous positive airway pressure was associated with a higher percentage of patients with neurological improvement one month after stroke compared to the control group (Rankin scale: 90.9% vs. 56.3%, P<0.01; Canadian scale: 88.2% vs. 72.7%, P<0.05, respectively). The cardiovascular mortality rate was 0% in patients treated with CPAP compared to 4.3% in the control group (P=0.16). The rate of cardiovascular events (cardiac ischemic events, stroke, and cardiovascular death) was 12.3% in the CPAP group and 11.6% in the conventional treatment group (P=0.56). The time from stroke onset to the first cardiovascular event was significantly longer in the CPAP group than in the control group (14.9 vs. 7.9 months, P=0.04); however, the cardiovascular event-free survival rate at two years was similar in both treatment arms, 87.7% in the CPAP group and 88.4% in the control group (P=0.91). Unfortunately, this study was only analyzed on a per-protocol and not on an intention-to-treat basis, thus 14 CPAP noncompliant patients were excluded from the analysis. As there were very few cardiovascular events in both groups during the follow-up time, the study was also underpowered to answer the question whether CPAP improves long-term vascular outcome in this setting.

In the randomized feasibility trial by Bravata and colleagues [48], 70 acute TIA patients were enrolled. Forty-five patients were randomized to the intervention arm (sleep study followed by CPAP treatment if OSA was present) and 25 to the control arm (sleep study only). At 90 days, vascular event rate (recurrent TIA, stroke, hospitalization for congestive heart failure, myocardial infarction, or death) tended to be highest (16%) among sleep apnea patients with no CPAP use, compared to 5% in patients with some CPAP use and 0% in patients with acceptable CPAP adherence (P=0.08). The preliminary findings of this pilot study support the hypothesis that CPAP may have a beneficial effect on cardiovascular events in patients with acute TIA. In a recently published study by the same authors, 55 patients with acute ischemic stroke were included; 31 patients were randomized to the intervention arm (sleep study followed by two days of CPAP that was continued for 30 days if OSA was present) and 24 patients to the control arm (sleep study only) [46]. At 30 days, patients allocated to the intervention group had greater improvements in the National Institutes of Health Stroke Scale (NIHSS) (−3.0) than control patients (−1.0) (P=0.03). Among patients with sleep apnea, greater improvement was observed with increasing CPAP use. However, the latter two studies were feasibility trials and thus not appropriately powered to definitely answer the question whether CPAP improves cerebrovascular outcome.

There is still urgent need for randomized controlled studies looking at the effect of CPAP treatment on cerebrovascular events in patients with OSA, without a history of previous stroke/TIA. In addition, appropriately powered randomized controlled trials investigating the impact of early CPAP intervention on vascular outcomes in patients with acute stroke/TIA are warranted. Such studies should be representative of a broad spectrum of stroke patients (e.g., severe stroke patients should possibly be included) and analyzed according to an intention-to-treat approach.

References

1. Sullivan CE, Berthon-Jones M, Issa FG et al. Reversal of obstructive sleep apnea by continuous positive airway pressure applied through the nares. *Lancet* 1981; **317**: 862–5.

2. Jenkinson C, Davies RJ, Mullins R, et al. Comparison of therapeutic and subtherapeutic nasal continuous positive airway pressure for obstructive sleep apnoea: a randomised prospective parallel trial. *Lancet* 1999; **353**: 2100–5.

3. Pepperell JCT, Ramdassingh-Dow S, Crosthwaite N, et al. Ambulatory blood pressure after therapeutic and subtherapeutic nasal continuous positive airway pressure for obstructive sleep apnoea: a randomised parallel trial. *Lancet* 2002; **359**: 204–10.

4. McArdle N, Devereux G, Heidarnejad H, et al. Long-term use of CPAP therapy for sleep apnea/hypopnea syndrome. *Am J Respir Crit Care Med* 1999; **159**: 1108–14.

5. Kohler M, Smith D, Tippett V, et al. Predictors of long-term compliance with continuous positive airway pressure. *Thorax* 2010; **65**: 829–32.

6. Bazzano LA, Khan Z, Reynolds K, et al. Effect of treatment with nocturnal nasal continuous positive airway pressure on blood pressure in patients with obstructive sleep apnea. *Hypertension* 2007; **50**: 417–23.

7. Kohler M, Ayers L, Pepperell JCT, et al. Effects of continuous positive airway pressure on systemic inflammation in patients with moderate to severe obstructive sleep apnoea: a randomised controlled trial. *Thorax* 2009; **64**: 67–73.

8. Kohler M, Pepperell JCT, Casadei B, et al. CPAP and measures of cardiovascular risk in males with OSAS. *Eur Respir J* 2008; **32**: 1488–96.

9. Kohler M, Stoewhas AC, Ayers L, et al. The effects of CPAP therapy withdrawal in patients with obstructive sleep apnoea: a randomized controlled trial. *Am J Respir Crit Care Med* 2011; **184**: 1192–9.

10. Peppard PE, Young T, Palta M, et al. Prospective study of the association between sleep-disordered breathing and hypertension. *N Engl J Med* 2000; **342**: 1378–84.

11. Alajmi M, Mulgrew AT, Fox J, et al. Impact of continuous positive airway pressure therapy on blood pressure in patients with obstructive sleep apnea hypopnea: a meta-analysis of randomized controlled trials. *Lung* 2007; **185**: 67–72.

12. Faccenda JF, Mackay TW, Boon NA, et al. Randomized placebo-controlled trial of continuous positive airway pressure on blood pressure in the sleep apnea-hypopnea syndrome. *Am J Respir Crit Care Med* 2001; **163**: 344–8.

13. Becker C, Jerrentrup A, Ploch T, et al. Effect of nasal continuous positive airway pressure treatment on BP in patients with obstructive sleep apnoea. *Circulation* 2003; **107**: 68–73.

14. Haentjens P, Van Meerhaeghe A, Moscariello A, et al. The impact of continuous positive airway pressure on blood pressure in patients with obstructive sleep apnea syndrome: evidence from a meta-analysis of placebo-controlled randomized trials. *Arch Intern Med* 2007; **167**: 757–64.

15. Alonso-Fernández A, Garcia-Río F, Arias MA, et al. Effects of CPAP on oxidative stress and nitrate efficiency in sleep apnoea: a randomised trial. *Thorax* 2009; **64**: 581–6.

16. Robinson GV, Langford BA, Smith DM, et al. Predictors of blood pressure fall with continuous positive airway pressure (CPAP) treatment of obstructive sleep apnoea (OSA). *Thorax* 2008; **63**: 855–9.

17. Barbe F, Duran-Cantolla J, Capote F, et al. Long-term effect of continuous positive airway pressure in hypertensive patients with sleep apnea. *Am J Respir Crit Care Med* 2010; **181**: 718–26.

18. Parati G, Valentini M. Do we need out-of-office blood pressure in every patient? *Curr Opin Cardiol* 2007; **22**: 321–8.

19. McDaid C, Duree KH, Griffin SC, et al. A systematic review of continuous positive airway pressure for obstructive sleep apnoea-hypopnoea syndrome. *Sleep Med Rev* 2009; **13**: 427–36.

20. Young T, Palta M, Dempsey J, et al. The occurence of sleep-disordered breathing among middle-aged adults. *N Engl J Med* 1993; **328**: 1230–5.

21. Robinson GV, Smith DM, Langford BA, et al. Continuous positive airway pressure does not reduce blood pressure in nonsleepy hypertensive OSA patients. *Eur Respir J* 2006; **27**: 1229–35.

22. Barbé F, Mayoralas LR, Duran J, et al. Treatment with continuous positive airway pressure is not effective in patients with sleep apnea but no daytime sleepiness: a randomized controlled trial. *Arch Intern Med* 2001; **134**: 1015–23.

23. Logan AG, Tkacova R, Perlikowski SM, et al. Refractory hypertension and sleep apnoea: effect of CPAP on blood pressure and baroreflex. *Eur Respir J* 2003; **21**: 241–7.

24. Ruttanaumpawan P, Nopmaneejumruslers C, Logan AG, et al. Association between refractory hypertension and obstructive sleep apnea. *J Hypertens* 2009; **27**: 1439–45.

25. Pedrosa RP, Drager LF, Gonzaga CC, et al. Obstructive sleep apnea: the most common secondary cause of hypertension associated with resistant hypertension. *Hypertension* 2011; **58**: 811–17.

26. Lozano L, Tovar JL, Sampol G, et al. Continuous positive airway pressure treatment in sleep apnea patients with resistant hypertension: a randomized controlled trial. *J Hypertens* 2010; **28**: 2161–8.

27. West SD, Nicoll DJ, Stradling JR. Prevalence of obstructive sleep apnoea in men with type 2 diabetes. *Thorax* 2006; **61**: 945–50.

28. West SD, Nicoll DJ, Wallace TM, et al. Effect of CPAP on insulin resistance and HbA1c in men with obstructive sleep apnoea and type 2 diabetes. *Thorax* 2007; **62**: 969–74.

29. Coughlin SR, Mawdsley L, Mugarza JA, et al. Cardiovascular and metabolic effects of CPAP in obese males with OSA. *Eur Respir J* 2007; **29**: 720–77.

30. Lam JC, Lam B, Yao TJ, et al. A randomised controlled trial of nasal continuous positive airway pressure on insulin sensitivity in obstructive sleep apnoea. *Eur Respir J* 2010; **35**: 138–45.

31. Donnan GA, Davis SM. Stroke and cholesterol: weakness of risk versus strength of therapy. *Stroke* 2004; **35**: 1526.

32. Corvol JC, Bouzamondo A, Sirol M, et al. Differential effects of lipid-lowering therapies on stroke prevention: a meta-analysis of randomized trials. *Arch Intern Med* 2003; **163**: 669–76.

33. Robinson GV, Pepperell JC, Segal HC, et al. Circulating cardiovascular risk factors in obstructive sleep apnoea: data from randomised controlled trials. *Thorax* 2004; **59**: 777–82.

34. Phillips CL, Yee BJ, Marshall NS, et al. Continuous positive airway pressure reduces postprandial lipidemia in obstructive sleep apnoea. *Am J Respir Crit Care Med* 2011; **184**: 355–61.

35. Hanly PJ, George CF, Millar TW, et al. Heart rate response to breath-hold, valsalva, and Mueller maneuvers in obstructive sleep apnea. *Chest* 1989; **95**: 735–9.

36. Linz D, Schotten U, Neuberger HR, et al. Negative tracheal pressure during obstructive respiratory events promotes atrial fibrillation by vagal activation. *Heart Rhythm* 2011; **8**: 1436–43.

37. Stoewhas AC, Namdar M, Biaggi P, et al. The effect of simulated obstructive apnea and hypopnea on aortic diameter and blood pressure. *Chest* 2011; **140**: 675–80.

38. Camen G, Clarenbach CF, Stoewhas AC, et al. The effect of simulated obstructive apnea and hypopnea on arrhythmic potential in healthy subjects. *Eur J Appl Physiol* 2012 [Epub ahead of print].

39. Ng CY, Liu T, Shehata M, et al. Meta-analysis of obstructive sleep apnea as predictor of atrial fibrillation recurrence after catheter ablation. *Am J Cardiol* 2011; **108**: 47–51.

40. Patel D, Mohanty P, Di Biase L, et al. Safety and efficacy of pulmonary vein antral isolation in patients with obstructive sleep apnea: the impact of continuous positive

airway pressure. *Circ Arrhythm Electrophysiol* 2010; **5**: 445–51.

41. Kanagala R, Murali NS, Friedman PA, et al. Obstructive sleep apnea and the recurrence of atrial fibrillation. *Circulation* 2003; **107**: 2589–94.

42. Arzt M, Young T, Finn L, et al. Association of sleep-disordered breathing and the occurrence of stroke. *Am J Respir Crit Care Med* 2005; **172**: 1447–51.

43. Redline S, Yenokyan G, Gottlieb DJ, et al. Obstructive sleep apnea-hypopnea and incident stroke. *Am J Respir Crit Care Med* 2010; **182**: 269–77.

44. Yaggi HK, Concato J, Kernan WN, et al. Obstructive sleep apnea as a risk factor for stroke and death. *N Engl J Med* 2005; **353**: 2034–41.

45. Parra O, Sánchez-Armengol A, Bonnin M, et al. Early treatment of obstructive apnoea and stroke outcome: a randomised controlled trial. *Eur Respir J* 2011; **37**: 1128–36.

46. Bravata DM, Concato J, Fried T, et al. Continuous positive airway pressure: evaluation of a novel therapy for patients with acute ischemic stroke. *Sleep* 2011; **34**: 1271–7.

47. Brown DL, Chervin RD, Kalbfleisch JD, et al. Sleep apnea treatment after stroke (SATS) trial: is it feasible? *J Stroke Cerebrovasc Dis* 2011 [Epub ahead of print].

48. Bravata DM, Concato J, Fried T, et al. Auto-titrating continuous positive airway pressure for patients with acute transient ischemic attack: a randomized feasibility trial. *Stroke* 2010; **41**: 1464–70.

49. Iranzo A, Santamaría J, Berenguer J, et al. Prevalence and clinical importance of sleep apnea in the first night after cerebral infarction. *Neurology* 2002; **58**: 911–16.

50. Foster GE, Hanly PJ, Ostrowski M, et al. Effects of continuous positive airway pressure on cerebral vascular response to hypoxia in patients with obstructive sleep apnea. *Am J Respir Crit Care Med* 2007; **175**: 720–5.

51. Martínez-García MA, Galiano-Blancart R, Román-Sánchez P, et al. Continuous positive airway pressure treatment in sleep apnea prevents new vascular events after ischemic stroke. *Chest* 2005; **128**: 2123–9.

52. Martínez-García MA, Soler-Cataluña JJ, Ejarque-Martínez L, et al. Continuous positive airway pressure treatment reduces mortality in patients with ischemic stroke and obstructive sleep apnea. *Am J Respir Crit Care Med* 2009; **180**: 36–41.

53. Martínez-García MA, Campos-Rodríguez F, Soler-Cataluña JJ, et al. Increased incidence of non-fatal cardiovascular events in stroke patients with sleep apnea. Effect of CPAP treatment. *Eur Respir J* 2012; **39**: 906–12.

Rehabilitation of stroke and sleep apnea

Behrouz Jafari and Vahid Mohsenin

Introduction

Each year in the United States, approximately 795 000 people experience a new or recurrent stroke; 137 000 of them will die from stroke complications [1]. On average, every four minutes, someone dies of a stroke. Of all strokes, 87% are ischemic, 10% are intracerebral hemorrhage, and 3% are subarachnoid hemorrhage strokes. Stroke is the third leading cause of death worldwide and more than 50% will have mental and physical impairment. One-third of stroke patients are under 65 years of age.

Obstructive sleep apnea syndrome is a highly prevalent disorder affecting 2%–4% of the general population in the United States. It is characterized by recurrent transient upper airway obstruction during sleep. Obstructive sleep apnea (OSA) results in oxygen desaturations and sleep fragmentation and increases the risk for cardiovascular disease including hypertension and stroke [2,3] and death [3,4].

Prevalence of obstructive sleep apnea in poststroke patients

Case-control studies

Clinical studies have shown that OSA is common among stroke patients, with a prevalence exceeding 50% (Table 11.1) [5,6]. Hudgel and coworkers performed polysomnography on eight patients if nocturnal finger pulse oximetry had suggested the presence of OSA one month after a unilateral cerebral ischemic or hemorrhagic stroke. In the stroke group with a mean age of 69 years, the apnea/hypopnea index (AHI) was 44 events/h compared to an AHI of 12 events/h in the control group with a mean age of 71 years [7].

Mohsenin and Valor prospectively studied 10 patients with unilateral hemispheric ischemic stroke with a mean age of 56 years, compared with 10 closely matched patients with a mean age of 52 years without stroke, in a rehabilitation unit. Polysomnographic studies were obtained within an average of three months of stroke occurrence. The prevalence of OSA with an AHI of >20 events/h was 80% in stroke patients and none in the control group [8].

In another study, 80 patients (mean age = 60 yr) with stroke (n=48) or transient ischemic attack (TIA) (n=32) were prospectively assessed for sleep-disordered breathing by polysomnography within a mean of nine days (range, 1–71 d) from TIA or stroke. Clinical and polysomnography data were compared with those of 25 healthy controls matched for age, gender, and body mass index (BMI). An AHI of ≥10 events/h was found in 62.5% of subjects and 12.5% of

---

Sleep, Stroke, and Cardiovascular Disease, ed. Antonio Culebras. Published by Cambridge University Press. © Cambridge University Press 2013.

Table 11.1. Case-control and cross-sectional studies of the prevalence of obstructive sleep apnea in patients with transient ischemic attacks and stroke

Study	Patients	Age	BMI	Frequency and characteristics of sleep-disordered breathing
Mohsenin et al., 1995 [8]	10 established stroke 10 controls	56±15 54±15	26.3±7.5 23.8±3.6	OSA in 80% of patients with hemispheric stroke, (AHI 52±30 events/h) None in controls (AHI 3±3 events/h)
Bassetti et al., 1999 [9]	48 stroke 32 TIA 25 controls	60±14 58±14 59±14	28.7±8.2 29.9±8.7 26.1±3.6	OSA in 62% of patients (AHI ≥10 events/h) as compared with 12% in 19 age- and gender-matched controls
Dyken et al., 1996 [10]	24 subacute stroke 27 controls	65±10 62±9	30.4±4.3 25.7±3.1	OSA in 71% of patients (AHI 18±22 events/h) as compared with 23% in controls(AHI 4±6 events/h)
Wessendorf et al., 2000 [14]	147 established stroke	61±10	29.2	OSA in 44% (AHI ≥10 events/h) and in 22% (AHI ≥20 events/h) of patients studied by 46±20 days after stroke
Parra et al., 2000 [15]	161 acute stroke	72±9	26.6±3.9	OSA in 71% (AHI ≥10 events/h) in 28% (AHI ≥30 events/h) within 48–72 h after stroke AHI ≥ 10 events/h in 62% (AHI ≥30 events/h in 20%) of patients 3 mo after stroke
Iranzo et al., 2002 [16]	50 acute stroke	67±10	26.3±3.9	OSA in 62% (AHI ≥10 events/h) and in 46% (AHI ≥20 events/h) with acute ischemic stroke
Turkington et al., 2002 [17]	120 acute stroke	79±10	23.6±4.0	OSA in 79% (AHI ≥5 events/h) and in 61% (AHI≥10 events/h) of patients within 24 h after stroke
Hui et al., 2002 [11]	51 acute stroke 25 controls	64±13 65±8	24.3±4.4 24.2±3.8	OSA in 49% (AHI ≥20 events/h) of stroke patients OSA in 25% (AHI ≥20 events/h) of controls
Harbison et al., 2002 [18]	68 subacute stroke	73±11	25.5±5.0	OSA in 94% (AHI ≥10 events/h) and in 66% (AHI ≥20 events/h) of patients within 2 wk of stroke AHI reduction from the acute to the subacute phase: 31±17 vs. 24±16, 6–9 wk after stroke
Disler et al., 2002 [33]	39 subacute stroke	65±15	NA	OSA in 50% (AHI >15 events/h) of patients 2 mo after stroke
McArdle et al., 2003 [12]	86 TIA 86 controls	65±11 66±10	27.0±5.0 27.0±5.0	OSA in 50% (AHI ≥15 events/h) of patients Mean AHI (21±17 events/h) similar to age- and gender-matched controls
Joo et al., 2011 [13]	61 acute stroke 13 TIA 64 controls	63±10 63±10 61±10	24.7±3.2 24.3±3.2 24.2±3.2	OSA in 51% (AHI 16±15 events/h) OSA in 69% (AHI 15±10 events/h) OSA in 32% (AHI 8±7 events/h)

TIA, transient ischemic attack; OSA, obstructive sleep apnea; AHI, apnea/hypopnea index.

controls. Between patients and controls there was a significant difference in the AHI (mean [range]: 28 [0–140] vs. 5 [0–24]; P<0.001) and nadir oxygen saturation (82% vs. 90%. P<0.001). Among the patients, frequency and severity of OSA were similar in stroke and TIA subjects [9].

Dyken and colleagues prospectively performed overnight polysomnography in 24 patients with a recent either ischemic or hemorrhagic stroke (13 men and 11 women; mean age of 65 yr) and 27 normal age- and gender-matched control subjects (13 men and 14 women; mean age of 62 yr) within approximately two to five weeks after each patient's stroke [10]. Obstructive sleep apnea was found in 77% of men with stroke compared with only 23% of male subjects without stroke (P=0.01). Likewise, 64% of women with stroke had OSA versus 14% of female subjects without stroke who had OSA (P=0.01). For men with stroke, the mean AHI was 22 events/h compared with 5 events/h (P=0.001). For women with stroke, the mean AHI was 32 events/h, while for female subjects without stroke it was 3 events/h (P=0.0024). Of note, these two studies also highlight the high prevalence of OSA in a non-stroke population with normal BMI.

In a case-control study, 67% of 23 women and 28 men within four days of stroke onset were found to have OSA with an AHI of ≥10 events/h and 49% with an AHI of ≥ 20 events/h compared to 24% of control subjects [11].

In view of the high prevalence of OSA in both the acute phase of stroke and established stroke, the question remained whether OSA preexisted prior to stroke or was a consequence of stroke, although there was no significant change in the AHI during the recovery from neurological impairment. This issue was explored by McArdle et al. in 86 carefully matched patients with TIA and 86 respective controls [12]. Because the neurological deficit in TIA is by definition transient, the presence of OSA in fully recovered post-TIA patients suggests OSA as a preexisting condition. Forty-nine of the 86 matched pairs were male and the BMI was similar among cases and controls. The primary outcome measure, the AHI, recorded during overnight polysomnography was the same for cases and controls (21events/h). Obstructive sleep apnea (AHI ≥15 events/h) was present in 50% of TIA and 60% of control subjects. However, the median number of 4% oxygen desaturations during sleep was slightly greater in the cases (12/h) than controls (6/h; P=0.04). The authors concluded that OSA does not appear to be strongly associated with TIA.

In a more recent study, Joo and colleagues compared patients with acute cerebral infarction with TIA and control subjects. Sixty-one patients with acute cerebral infarction and 13 patients with TIA were consecutively enrolled. Sleep-disordered breathing was evaluated within 48 h of stroke or TIA onset using a portable screening device. Sixty-four age-matched patients' spouses or family members with no history of physician-diagnosed stroke were enrolled as controls. The prevalence of OSA was 50.8% in acute cerebral infarction patients, 69.2% in TIA, and 32.8% in controls. The AHI was significantly higher in patients with acute cerebral infarction (15.6±14.7 events/h) and TIA (14.6±10.4 events/h) than in the controls (7.8±7.0 events/h; P=0.001). The BMI and systolic blood pressure (SBP) were significantly higher in patients with OSA than in those without OSA. Multiple logistic regression analysis showed that BMI (odds ratio, 1.293; P=0.027) and SBP (odds ratio, 1.030; P=0.004) were found to independently predict OSA in patients with acute cerebral infarction and TIA [13].

Cross-sectional studies

A cross-sectional study performing polysomnography on 147 consecutive patients (95 men, 52 women, aged 61±10 yr) with first-ever stroke, in a rehabilitation center, showed the presence of OSA with an AHI of >10 events/h in 44% and an AHI of >20 events/h in 22% of the patients. Polysomnography was performed 46±20 days after stroke and showed primarily obstructive apneas. As in previously mentioned studies, subjective sleepiness was not a prominent symptom even in those with severe OSA. Central apnea as the predominant form of sleep-disordered breathing was seen in only 6% of patients. The prevalence of hypertension and coronary heart disease were higher among stroke patients with an AHI of 20 events/h or higher than in those without sleep-disordered breathing [14].

In a study examining the relationship between topographical patterns of stroke with sleep-disordered breathing, Parra et al. [15] prospectively studied 161 consecutive patients admitted to a stroke unit. A portable respiratory recording study was performed within 48–72 h after admission (acute phase), and subsequently after three months (stable phase). During the acute phase, 116 patients (72%) had an AHI of >10 events/h and 45 (28%) had an AHI of >30 events/h. No relationships were found between sleep-related respiratory events and the topographical parenchymatous location of the neuro-logical lesion or vascular involvement. Cheyne–Stokes breathing was observed in 42 cases (26.1%). There were no significant differences in sleep apnea according to the stroke subtype except for the central apnea index (CAI). During the stable phase a second portable respiratory recording was performed in 86 patients: 62% had an AHI of >10 events/h and 20% had an AHI of >30 events/h. The CAI was significantly lower than that in those in the acute phase (3.3 vs. 6.2, respectively) ($P<0.05$) while the obstructive apnea index remained unchanged.

The prevalence of sleep apnea during the first night after hemispheric ischemic stroke was investigated in 50 patients by undergoing polysomnography within 24 hours of stroke onset. There were 30 males and 20 females with a mean age of 66.8±9.5 years. Thirty-one (62%) subjects had OSA (AHI ≥10 events/h). Of these, 23 (46% of the cohort) had an AHI of >20 events/h and 21 (42% of the cohort) an AHI of ≥25 events/h. Sleep-related stroke onset occurred in 24 (48% of all the patients) patients and was predicted only by an AHI of ≥25 events/h on logistic regression analysis. Obstructive sleep apnea was related to early neuro-logical worsening and oxyhemoglobin desaturations but not to sleep history before stroke onset, infarct topography and size, neurological severity, or functional outcome. Early neurological worsening was found in 15 (30%) patients, and logistic regression analysis identified OSA and serum glucose as its independent predictors [16].

Turkington and colleagues confirmed these findings in 120 patients with stroke within 24 hours of stroke onset and again showed a high prevalence of OSA in these patients. They found that 79%, 61%, and 45% of the patients had an AHI greater than 5, 10, and 15 events/h, respectively. Obstructive sleep apnea tended to be position-dependent with higher AHI in the supine position. On logistic regression analysis, BMI ($P=0.025$), neck circumference ($P=0.026$), and limb weakness ($P=0.025$) independently predicted the occurrence of OSA in the first 24 hours after acute stroke [17].

In a prospective uncontrolled observational study, Harbison et al. performed respiratory sleep studies at week 2 from stroke onset in 68 patients; 94% of patients had an AHI of ≥10 events/h with a mean AHI of 30 events/h. The mean AHI was higher in subjects with lacunar compared with cortical strokes (44 vs. 28 events/h; $P<0.05$), in subjects aged ≥65 years (32 vs. 21 events/h; $P<0.05$). In 50 paired studies, the mean AHI fell from 31 to 24 events/h ($P<0.01$) and the proportion with an AHI of ≥10 events/h fell from 96% to 72%. Although there was a statistically significant decrease in the AHI between week 2 and weeks 6–9 from stroke onset, a clinically meaningful OSA remained highly prevalent [18].

As part of the Sleep Heart Health Study, Shahar et al. examined the cross-sectional association between sleep-disordered breathing and self-reported cardiovascular disease in 6424 free-living individuals who underwent overnight, unattended polysomnography at home. In this community-dwelling general population, mild to moderate disordered breathing during sleep was highly prevalent with a median AHI of 4.4 events/h (interquartile range: 1.3–11.0). A total of 1023 participants (16%) reported at least one manifestation of cardiovascular disease (myocardial infarction, angina, coronary revascularization procedure, heart failure, or stroke). The multivariable-adjusted relative odds (95% CI) of prevalent cardiovascular disease for the second, third, and fourth quartiles of the AHI (versus the first) were 0.98 (0.77–1.24), 1.28 (1.02–1.61), and 1.42 (1.13–1.78), respectively. Sleep-disordered breathing was associated more strongly with self-reported heart failure and stroke than with self-reported coronary heart disease. These findings show that the presence of mild to moderate OSA has an influence on manifestations of cardiovascular disease in the general population [19].

Association between obstructive sleep apnea and stroke

These studies suggested that OSA may have existed before the stroke. However, a cause-and-effect relationship cannot be established without prospective controlled studies to determine the incident rate of stroke or TIA in patients with and without OSA.

Prospective longitudinal studies

Previous studies have suggested that OSA may be an important risk factor for stroke. It has not been determined, however, whether the OSA is independently related to the risk of stroke or death from any cause after adjustment for other risk factors, including hypertension. In a large observational cohort study [3] consecutive patients from a university sleep medicine center underwent nocturnal polysomnography, and subsequent events (strokes and deaths) were verified over the ensuing six years. The diagnosis of OSA was based on an AHI of ≥5 events/h; patients with an AHI of <5 events/h served as the comparison group. Among 1022 enrolled patients, 697 (68%) had OSA. At baseline, the mean AHI in the patients with OSA was 35 events/h, as compared with a mean AHI of 2 events/h in the comparison group. Incident stroke or death from any cause (22 strokes, 50 deaths) occurred in 88 patients (9%) at a rate of 3.48 events per 100 person–years, as compared with 4.9% in the comparison group (2 strokes and 14 deaths; 1.60 events per 100 person–years). The groups were closely matched for traditional stroke risk factors. Proportional-hazards analysis was used to determine the independent effect of OSA on the composite outcome of stroke or death from any cause. After adjustment for age, gender, race, smoking status, alcohol-consumption status, BMI, and the presence or absence of diabetes mellitus, hyperlipidemia, atrial fibrillation, and hypertension, OSA retained a statistically significant association with stroke or death (hazard ratio, 1.97; 95% CI, 1.12–3.48; P=0.01). In a trend analysis, increased severity of sleep apnea at baseline was associated with an increased risk of the development of the composite end point (P=0.005). When the highest AHI quartile (AHI >36 events/h) was compared with the lowest quartile (AHI ≤3 events/h), the hazard ratio was 3.3 (95% CI, 1.74–6.26). The authors concluded that OSA significantly increases the risk of stroke or death from any cause, and the increase is independent of traditional cardiovascular risk factors, including hypertension.

A similar study was conducted in a general population drawn from the Wisconsin Sleep Cohort Study, with stroke alone as the outcome of interest [2]. From this cohort, 1189 subjects were followed for four years after undergoing an attended polysomnography. In the subgroups of participants with an AHI of <5, 5 to less than 20, and ≥20 events/h, the incidence of strokes was 1.33, 0.54, and 5.75 per 100 person–years, respectively. Obstructive sleep apnea with an AHI of ≥20 events/h was associated with an increased risk of suffering a first-ever stroke over the next four years (unadjusted odds ratio, 4.31; 95% CI, 1.31–14.15; P=0.02). However, after adjustment for age, gender, and BMI, the odds ratio was still elevated, but was no longer significant (3.08; 95% CI, 0.74–12.81; P=0.12). This odds ratio is comparable to that in the study by Yaggi et al. on the sleep clinic population as previously discussed [3]. However, despite similar effect size and because of the nature of the general population with a wider confidence interval, the statistical significance was attenuated [2].

The risk of stroke in the general population in relationship to OSA was further investigated in the Sleep Heart Health Study cohort, which is a community-based, prospective cohort study of the cardiovascular consequences of OSA. The characterization of the cohort at baseline took place in the 1995–1998 period and included overnight unattended polysomnography. The data for this study were collected prospectively through 2006, with a median of 8.7 years (interquartile range 7.8–9.4 yr) of follow-up. The primary exposure was the OSA-related AHI and outcome was incident ischemic stroke. A total of 5422 participants without a history of stroke at the baseline examination and untreated for sleep apnea were followed for a median of 8.7 years. One hundred and ninety-three ischemic strokes were observed. In covariate-adjusted Cox proportional hazard models, a significant positive association between ischemic stroke and AHI was observed in men (P value for linear trend: P=0.016), as shown by a Kaplan-Meier stroke-free survival curve in Figure 11.1. Men in the highest AHI quartile (>19 events/h) had an adjusted hazard ratio of 2.86 (95% CI, 1.1–7.4). In the mild to moderate range (AHI, 5–25 events/h), each one-unit increase in

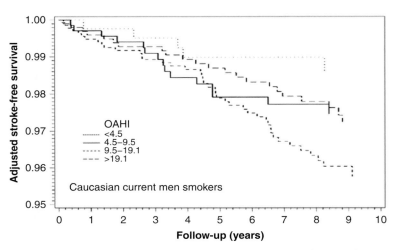

Figure 11.1. Adjusted Kaplan-Meier stroke-free survival estimated as a function of the obstructive apnea/hypopnea index (AHI) quartiles. This study of men smokers shows that the more severe the OSA the higher the risk of stroke over a median of 8.6 years. Adapted from Redline et al. [20].

AHI in men was estimated to increase stroke risk by 6% (95% CI, 2%–10%). In women, stroke was not significantly associated with AHI quartiles, but increased risk was observed at an AHI of >25 events/h. This large prospective population-based study replicates prior studies on the general population and clinic patients, supporting the causal link between OSA and stroke [20].

Sahlin and coworkers investigated whether obstructive or central sleep apnea was related to shorter long-term survival among patients with stroke. Of 151 patients admitted for in-hospital stroke rehabilitation, 132 (aged 77.5±7.1 years) underwent overnight sleep apnea recordings at a mean of 23±8 days after the onset of stroke. All patients were followed up prospectively for a mean of 10.0±0.6 years, with death as the primary outcome. Obstructive sleep apnea was defined when the AHI was ≥15 events/h, and CSA was defined when the central AHI was ≥15 events/h. Patients with obstructive and central AHI of <15 events/h served as control subjects. Of 132 enrolled patients, 116 (88%) had died at follow-up. The causes of death were regarded as cardiovascular in 74.0%, cancer in 9.9%, other causes in 14.3%, and unknown in 1.8%. The risk of death was higher among the 23 patients with OSA than the controls (adjusted hazard ratio, 1.76; 95% CI, 1.05–2.95; P=0.03), independent of age, gender, BMI, smoking, hypertension, diabetes mellitus, atrial fibrillation, Mini-Mental State Examination score, and Barthel index of activities of daily living (ADL). There was no difference in mortality between the 28 patients with central sleep apnea and the controls (adjusted hazard ratio, 1.07; 95% CI, 0.65–1.76; P=0.80). Patients with stroke and OSA had an increased risk of early death. Central sleep apnea was not related to early death among these patients [4].

Effect of obstructive sleep apnea on neurological impairment after stroke

The presence of OSA in the setting of stroke is associated with an unfavorable clinical course, including early neurological worsening, delirium, depressed mood, impaired functional capacity and cognition, longer period of hospitalization and rehabilitation, and increased mortality.

Good et al. examined the effect of OSA on neurological recovery in 47 patients with recent ischemic stroke (a median of 13 days from stroke onset). Medical history, sleep history, location of stroke, and severity of neurological deficit were recorded. Functional abilities were measured with the use of the Barthel index. Outcome variables included ability to return home at discharge, continued residence at home at 3 and 12 months, Barthel index at discharge and at 3 and 12 months, and death from any cause at 12 months. The oxygen desaturation index (ODI, number of desaturation events per hour of recording time) was 9.5±9.7 events/h, with 32% having an ODI of >10 events/h. Eighteen of 19 patients (95%) who underwent polysomnography had an AHI of >10 events/h and 53% had an AHI of >30 events/h. Oximetry measures of OSA correlated with lower Barthel index scores at discharge and a lower Barthel index at 3- and 12-month follow-ups (P≤0.05, Pearson coefficients). Oximetry measures correlated with the return home after discharge, but the association between oximetry measures and living at home was lost at 12 months [21].

Fifty patients with hemispheric stroke were evaluated with polysomnography on admission and assessed by the Scandinavian stroke scale and outcome by the Barthel index on the third day, at discharge, and at one, three, and six months. Of these patients, 62% had OSA (AHI ≥ 10 events/h). The OSA was related to early neurological worsening and oxyhemoglobin desaturations but not to sleep history before stroke onset, infarct topography and size, neurological severity, or functional outcome. Early neurological worsening was found in 30% of patients, and logistic regression analysis identified OSA as an independent predictor of early neurological worsening but not of functional outcome at six months [16].

Sandberg et al. investigated the presence of OSA after stroke and its relationship to delirium, depressed mood, cognitive functioning, ability to perform ADL, and psychiatric and behavioral symptoms. One hundred and thirty-three patients (78 women and 55 men, mean age, 77.1±7.7 yr) consecutively admitted to a geriatric stroke rehabilitation unit underwent overnight respiratory sleep recordings at 23±7 days (range, 11–41 d) after suffering a stroke. The patients were assessed using the organic brain syndrome scale, Montgomery-Asberg depression rating scale, mini-mental state examination (MMSE), and Barthel-ADL index. Obstructive sleep apnea was defined as an AHI of ≥10 events/h. Fifty-nine percent of patients had OSA. More patients with OSA than without were delirious, depressed, or more ADL-dependent. Multivariate analysis showed that OSA was associated with delirium, depressed mood, latency in reaction and in response to verbal stimuli, and impaired ADL-ability [22].

Sixty-one stroke patients admitted to a stroke rehabilitation unit underwent polysomnography (45±24 days from stroke onset) and evaluation using the Functional Independence Measure. Obstructive sleep apnea was found in 60% of patients (AHI ≥10 events/h), while 12% predominantly had central sleep apnea. Although the severity of stroke was similar in the two groups, those with sleep apnea had lower functional capacity (80.2±3.6 vs. 94.7±4.3; P<0.05 at admission, and 101.5±2.8 vs. 112.9±2.7; P < 0.05 at discharge) and spent significantly more days in rehabilitation (45.5±2.3 vs. 32.1±2.7 d; P<0.005). In addition, multiple regression analysis showed that OSA was significantly and independently related to functional impairment and length of hospitalization [23].

In a prospective study, 30 first-ever stroke patients underwent continuous overnight pulse oximetry during sleep for the presence of desaturation events (a fall of arterial saturation of >4% from the baseline). The respiratory disturbance index (RDI) was defined as the number of desaturations per hour of sleep. Functional assessment was done at admission and at discharge using the functional independence measure instrument. After adjusting for admission functional status, the RDI was negatively correlated with the functional gain on linear regression, explaining 20.9% of the total variance [24].

Sixty consecutively enrolled Chinese patients with stroke were evaluated at three and six months after stroke onset by the Barthel index and the Scandinavian stroke scale. Sixty-five percent had OSA with an AHI of ≥5 events/h. On logistic regression analysis, the Scandinavian stroke scale on admission (odds ratio 0.74; 95% CI, 0.62–0.88; P=0.001) and the AHI (odds ratio 1.09; 95% CI, 1.02–1.17; P<0.05) independently predicted poor functional outcome on the Barthel index at three months. At six months, the Barthel index was predicted only by the Scandinavian stroke scale (odds ratio 0.83, 95% CI, 0.74–0.92; P=0.001) [25].

These studies demonstrate a high prevalence of OSA at different time points from stroke onset. Obstructive sleep apnea exerts a negative effect on the functional recovery of these patients. The frequency of OSA remains unchanged despite neurological recovery, indicating the presence of OSA pre-dating the stroke. Therefore, patients with stroke should be screened early for OSA and treated. However, the question remains whether early intervention for the treatment of OSA shortly after stroke onset will alter the neurological recovery.

Effects of early treatment of obstructive sleep apnea in stroke rehabilitation and outcome

The central nervous system during stroke-in-progress or hours poststroke is susceptible to further ischemia and tissue injury due to loss of cerebral autoregulation and tissue hypoxia. The fluctuations in SBP and intermittent hypoxemia accompanying OSA can impair blood supply and oxygen to the penumbra surrounding the ischemic and infarcted zones, increasing the probability of further tissue damage [26,27]. Prospective observational studies in the general population and clinical samples have shown that stroke is indeed the consequence rather than the cause of OSA. Sleep apnea, in the setting of an acute stroke, may be associated with early neurological worsening, decreased functional recovery, and increased mortality. Patients with TIA are at increased risk of recurrent vascular events; 25% of TIA patients will have a cerebro- or cardiovascular event or death in the 90 days after TIA, and over the long term, 11% per year will have a stroke, myocardial infarction, or vascular death. Half of the recurrent events occur in the first two days after TIA. In general, interventions aimed at improving poststroke functioning are more effective the earlier they are delivered after symptom onset. With the advent of portable polysomnography and autoadjusting continuous positive airway pressure (auto-CPAP) devices, it is possible to diagnose and treat obstructive OSA during the acute phase of stroke and TIA.

One hundred and five poststroke patients (average of 60 days from stroke) in a rehabilitation unit underwent polysomnography followed by auto-CPAP treatment. There was an 80% reduction of respiratory events with concomitant increase in oxygen saturation and improvement in sleep architecture. No serious side-effects were noticed. Seventy-four patients (70.5%) continued treatment at home. Non-acceptance was associated with a lower functional status, as measured by the Barthel index, and the presence of aphasia. Ten days after initiation of auto-CPAP, compliant users showed a clear improvement in wellbeing versus noncompliant patients. Only the compliant group had a reduction in mean nocturnal blood pressure (diastolic BP, -8±7.3 mmHg vs. 0.8±8.4 mmHg; $P=0.037$) [28].

In an uncontrolled prospective study of patients two months after stroke, the subjects underwent respiratory polygraphy and those with an AHI of >20 events/h were offered CPAP treatment. Those that could not tolerate CPAP were followed as a comparison group. During the 18 months of follow-up, the CPAP-compliant group had a significantly lower incident rate of new stroke (6.7%) compared with the noncompliant group (36.1%; long-rank, P=0.03) [29].

In a randomized, open-label, parallel group trial of CPAP within three weeks of stroke onset, 22 patients received CPAP for four weeks and 22 patients served as controls participating in a similar rehabilitation program without CPAP. The primary outcomes were the Canadian neurological scale, six-minute walk test distance, sustained attention response test, and the digit or spatial span-backward. Secondary outcomes included Epworth sleepiness scale, Stanford sleepiness scale, functional independence measure, Chedoke McMaster stroke assessment, cognitive function, and Beck depression inventory. These assessments were done blinded to the CPAP treatment. The CPAP group experienced improvement in stroke-related impairment (Canadian neurological scale score, P<0.001) but not in the six-minute walk test distance, sustained attention response test, or digit or spatial span-backward. Regarding secondary outcomes, the CPAP group experienced improvements in the Epworth sleepiness scale (P<0.001), motor component of the functional independence measure (P=0.05), Chedoke-McMaster stroke assessment of upper and lower limb motor recovery test of the leg (P=0.001), and the affective component of depression (P=0.006), but not cognitive function [30].

Previous studies have examined the feasibility and potential beneficial effects of OSA treatment on neurological and cognitive functions of patients during the stable phase of stroke, in a rehabilitation setting. However, a significant part of brain structural damage and functional impairment occur early in the course of the stroke. Any intervention for improving the chances of recovery and prevention of further injury should take place early. The collaborative group of investigators at Yale and the University of Iowa studied the feasibility and effectiveness of CPAP in patients with acute stroke and TIA with OSA. Stroke patients were randomized to an intervention group (stroke standard of care plus auto-CPAP) and control group (only stroke standard of care). Stroke patients randomized to the intervention group received two nights of auto-CPAP, but only those with evidence of OSA received auto-CPAP for the remainder of the 30-day period. Intervention patients received polysomnography 30 days poststroke. Control patients received polysomnography at baseline and after 30 days. Acceptable auto-CPAP adherence was defined as ≥4 h/night for ≥75% nights. Change in stroke severity was assessed comparing the National Institute of Health stroke scale (NIHSS) at baseline with that at 30 days. The two groups (intervention n=31, control n=24) had similar baseline stroke severity (both with a median NIHSS of 3.0). Among patients with complete polysomnography data, the majority had OSA: baseline: 13/15 (86.7%) control patients; 30 days: 24/35 (68.6%) control and intervention patients. Intervention patients had greater improvements in the NIHSS (−3.0) than control patients (−1.0) (P=0.03). Among patients with OSA, greater improvement was observed with increasing auto-CPAP use: −1.0 for control patients not using auto-CPAP, −2.5 for intervention patients with some auto-CPAP use, and −3.0 for intervention patients with acceptable auto-CPAP adherence. Auto-CPAP was well tolerated by patients during the acute phase of their stroke and appeared to improve neurological recovery from stroke [31]. A similar study on TIA patients by the same group showed that CPAP administration in TIA patients is feasible [32]. Larger studies are needed to evaluate whether a strategy of diagnosing and treating OSA early can reduce recurrent vascular events after TIA and stroke.

Conclusion

Several cohort studies have demonstrated that OSA significantly increases the risk of stroke independent of potential confounding risk factors. This is particularly important, given that OSA is a potentially modifiable risk factor. Randomized controlled trials of CPAP in OSA patients with follow-up of cerebro- and cardiovascular outcomes suggest a clinically significant risk reduction associated with the use of CPAP. In view of the potential benefits of airway pressurization on prognosis and functional outcome with improving the quality of life and cognitive function, and the effect on acceleration of recovery in the rehabilitation of patients with stroke, clinicians should have a low threshold for evaluating symptoms of sleep-disordered breathing in their patients. Interventions aimed at improving poststroke functioning are more effective if delivered early after stroke symptom onset.

References

1. Lloyd-Jones D, Adams RJ, Brown TM, et al. Heart disease and stroke statistics – 2010 update: a report from the American Heart Association. *Circulation* 2010; **121**: e46–e215.

2. Arzt M, Young T, Finn L, et al. Association of sleep-disordered breathing and the occurrence of stroke. *Am J Respir Crit Care Med* 2005; **172**: 1447–51.

3. Yaggi HK, Concato J, Kernan WN, et al. Obstructive sleep apnea as a risk factor for stroke and death. *N Engl J Med* 2005; **353**: 2034–41.

4. Sahlin C, Sandberg O, Gustafson Y, et al. Obstructive sleep apnea is a risk factor for death in patients with stroke: a 10-year follow-up. *Arch Intern Med* 2008; **168**: 297–301.

5. Dyken ME, Im KB. Obstructive sleep apnea and stroke. *Chest* 2009; **136**: 1668–77.

6. Yaggi H, Mohsenin V. Obstructive sleep apnoea and stroke. *Lancet Neurol* 2004; **3**: 333–42.

7. Hudgel DW, Devadatta P, Quadri M, et al. Mechanism of sleep-induced periodic breathing in convalescing stroke patients and healthy elderly subjects. *Chest* 1993; **104**: 1503–10.

8. Mohsenin V, Valor R. Sleep apnea in patients with hemispheric stroke. *Arch Phys Med Rehabil* 1995; **76**: 71–6.

9. Bassetti C, Aldrich MS. Sleep apnea in acute cerebrovascular diseases: final report on 128 patients. *Sleep* 1999; **22**: 217–23.

10. Dyken ME, Somers VK, Yamada T, et al. Investigating the relationship between stroke and obstructive sleep apnea. *Stroke* 1996; **27**: 401–7.

11. Hui DS, Choy DK, Wong LK, et al. Prevalence of sleep-disordered breathing and continuous positive airway pressure compliance: results in Chinese patients with first-ever ischemic stroke. *Chest* 2002; **122**: 852–60.

12. McArdle N, Riha RL, Vennelle M, et al. Sleep-disordered breathing as a risk factor for cerebrovascular disease: a case-control study in patients with transient ischemic attacks. *Stroke* 2003; **34**: 2916–21.

13. Joo BE, Seok HY, Yu SW, et al. Prevalence of sleep-disordered breathing in acute ischemic stroke as determined using a portable sleep apnea monitoring device in Korean subjects. *Sleep Breath* 2011; **15**: 77–82.

14. Wessendorf TE, Teschler H, Wang YM, et al. Sleep-disordered breathing among patients with first-ever stroke. *J Neurol* 2000; **247**: 41–7.

15. Parra O, Arboix A, Bechich S, et al. Time course of sleep-related breathing disorders in first-ever stroke or transient ischemic attack. *Am J Respir Crit Care Med* 2000; **161**: 375–80.

16. Iranzo A, Santamaria J, Berenguer J, et al. Prevalence and clinical importance of sleep apnea in the first night after cerebral infarction. *Neurology* 2002; **58**: 911–16.

17. Turkington PM, Bamford J, Wanklyn P, et al. Prevalence and predictors of upper airway obstruction in the first 24 hours after acute stroke. *Stroke* 2002; **33**: 2037–42.

18. Harbison J, Ford GA, James OF, et al. Sleep-disordered breathing following acute stroke. *QJM* 2002; **95**: 741–7.

19. Shahar E, Whitney CW, Redline S, et al. Sleep-disordered breathing and cardiovascular disease: cross-sectional results of the Sleep Heart Health Study. *Am J Respir Crit Care Med* 2001; **163**: 19–25.

20. Redline S, Yenokyan G, Gottlieb DJ, et al. Obstructive sleep apnea-hypopnea and incident stroke: the Sleep Heart Health Study. *Am J Respir Crit Care Med* 2010; **182**: 269–77.

21. Good DC, Henkle JQ, Gelber D, et al. Sleep-disordered breathing and poor functional outcome after stroke. *Stroke* 1996; **27**: 252–9.

22. Sandberg O, Franklin KA, Bucht G, et al. Sleep apnea, delirium, depressed mood, cognition, and ADL ability after stroke. *J Am Geriatr Soc* 2001; **49**: 391–7.

23. Kaneko Y, Hajek VE, Zivanovic V, et al. Relationship of sleep apnea to functional capacity and length of hospitalization following stroke. *Sleep* 2003; **26**: 293–7.

24. Cherkassky T, Oksenberg A, Froom P, et al. Sleep-related breathing disorders and

rehabilitation outcome of stroke patients: a prospective study. *Am J Phys Med Rehabil* 2003; **82**: 452–5.

25. Yan-fang S, Yu-ping W. Sleep-disordered breathing: impact on functional outcome of ischemic stroke patients. *Sleep Med* 2009; **10**: 717–19.

26. Balfors EM, Franklin KA. Impairment of cerebral perfusion during obstructive sleep apneas. *Am J Respir Crit Care Med* 1994; **150**: 1587–91.

27. Urbano F, Roux F, Schindler J, et al. Impaired cerebral autoregulation in obstructive sleep apnea. *J Appl Physiol* 2008; **105**: 1852–7.

28. Wessendorf TE, Wang YM, Thilmann AF, et al. Treatment of obstructive sleep apnoea with nasal continuous positive airway pressure in stroke. *Eur Respir J* 2001; **18**: 623–9.

29. Martinez-Garcia MA, Galiano-Blancart R, Roman-Sanchez P, et al. Continuous positive airway pressure treatment in sleep apnea prevents new vascular events after ischemic stroke. *Chest* 2005; **128**: 2123–9.

30. Ryan CM, Bayley M, Green R, et al. Influence of continuous positive airway pressure on outcomes of rehabilitation in stroke patients with obstructive sleep apnea. *Stroke* 2011; **42**: 1062–7.

31. Bravata DM, Concato J, Fried T, et al. Continuous positive airway pressure: evaluation of a novel therapy for patients with acute ischemic stroke. *Sleep* 2011; **34**: 1271–7.

32. Bravata DM, Concato J, Fried T, et al. Auto-titrating continuous positive airway pressure for patients with acute transient ischemic attack: a randomized feasibility trial. *Stroke* 2010; **41**: 1464–70.

33. Disler P, Hansford A, Skelton J, et al. Diagnosis and treatment of obstructive sleep apnea in a stroke rehabilitation unit: a feasibility study. *Am J Phys Med Rehabil* 2002; **81**: 622–5.

Restless legs syndrome, periodic limb movements in sleep, and vascular risk factors

Federica Provini

Introduction

Restless legs syndrome (RLS) is a very common sensorimotor disorder usually associated with unpleasant sensations and characterized by an irresistible desire to move the legs [1]. Symptoms occur during periods of rest, such as sitting or lying down, and are partially or totally relieved by movement. Restless legs syndrome worsens in the evening and night, delaying sleep onset and/or causing frequent awakenings, especially during the first part of nocturnal sleep [1]. A variable RLS prevalence rate has been reported ranging from 4% to 29% of the general adult population, making it one of the most common sleep disorders [2,3]. Even the studies reporting lower prevalences suggest that close to 1 in 100 persons suffers from RLS that seriously impacts on quality of life, while 1 in 25 have symptoms causing at least some degree of distress.

About 80%–90% of RLS patients also experience periodic limb movements (PLM) of sleep (PLMS). Periodic limb movements are involuntary, repetitive, and stereotyped short-lasting movements of the lower and sometimes upper limbs, often consisting of a dorsiflexion of the big toe with fanning of the small toes, accompanied by flexion at the ankles, knees, and thighs. Each movement lasts 0.5–10 s and recurs at intervals of 5–90 s, in a series of at least four such movements in sequence that are at least 8 μV in amplitude with a remarkable periodicity of approximately 20–40 s [4] (Figures 12.1 and Figures 12.2).

The severity of PLMS is scored by the PLM index (i.e., number of movements per hour of sleep). Periodic limb movements of sleep are most frequent during non-rapid eye movement (NREM) sleep stages 1 and 2 and are maximally suppressed during REM sleep. In patients in whom PLMS are found during sleep, especially in RLS, PLM of the same type may occur during quiet wakefulness, before sleep onset, or in the course of nocturnal waking episodes, and have been called periodic limb movements while awake (PLMW). An overnight PLM index of 15 in adults is considered pathological [5].

In the last ten years, a growing body of literature suggests an association between RLS, hypertension, and cardiovascular diseases (CVD) [3]. Recent epidemiological studies suggest that RLS with PLMS may also lead to stroke. However, the cause–effect link remains controversial because, although RLS/PLMS may lead to stroke, it is also possible that stroke may lead to RLS/PLMS [6,7].

An increased cardio- and cerebrovascular risk was also documented in patients with chronic kidney disease and a higher PLMS index [8–10]. A recent 18-month prospective

Sleep, Stroke, and Cardiovascular Disease, ed. Antonio Culebras. Published by Cambridge University Press. © Cambridge University Press 2013.

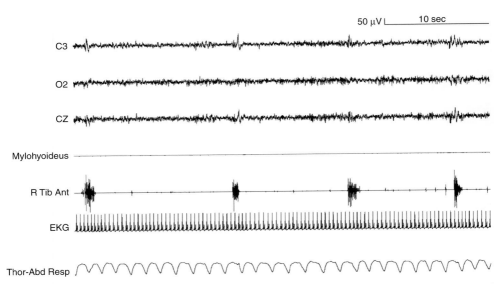

Figure 12.1. Polygraphic recording of periodic limb movements during stage 2 non-rapid eye movement (NREM) sleep. Elecromyographic bursts on the right tibialis anterior muscle (R Tib Ant) are seen recurring periodically every 15–20 seconds. EKG, electrocardiogram; Thor-Abd Resp, thoracoabdominal respirogram.

observational study of one hundred end-stage kidney disease patients on dialysis found that RLS affected 31% of the study population. During observation, 47% of patients experienced new cardiovascular events (64.5% with and 39.1% without RLS; P=0.019), and new cardiovascular events increased with the severity of RLS. Mortality was 20% in all patients; 32.3% in those with, and 14.5% in patients without RLS (P=0.04) [10].

While the temporal/causal relationship between RLS and cardiovascular disease and related disorders remains unclear due to sparse prospective data, several non-mutually exclusive mechanisms are possible in determining a higher cardiovascular risk in the RLS population.

The autonomic activation caused by repeated autonomic arousals associated with PLMS, a hypothalamic–pituitary–adrenal (HPA) axis dysregulation along with sleep loss, mood disturbance, and unhealthy lifestyle factors, or the presence of common risk factors for heart disease and RLS, such as diabetes, are all possible causes predisposing RLS patients to CVD.

This chapter examines the evidence from recent studies linking RLS to increased risk for the subsequent development and progression of CVD and discusses the possible causal pathways of this association.

Association of restless legs syndrome, hypertension, and cardiovascular diseases: epidemiology

Some studies support a positive relationship between RLS and hypertension, even after adjustment for confounding factors such as body mass index (BMI), smoking, and other sleep disorders [11–15], whereas other studies have failed to establish any relationship [3,16–21] (Table 12.1). More than 10 large population-based studies from nine countries provided information on the association between RLS and CVD [3,12,21–24].

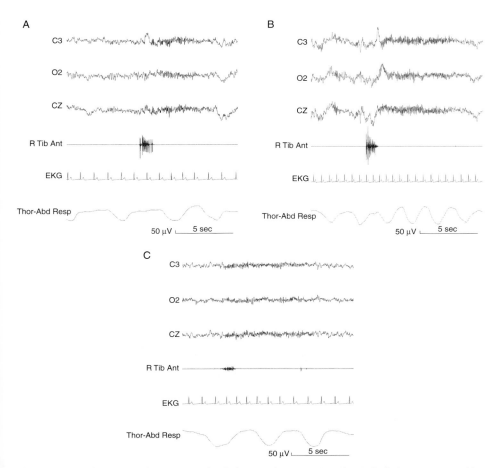

Figure 12.2. Polysomnographic segments (A–C) showing the association of periodic limb movements with an electroencephalographic (EEG) arousal. R Tib Ant, right tibialis anterior muscle; EKG, electrocardiogram; Thor-Abd Resp, thoracoabdominal respirogram.

Ulfberg et al. conducted a study on a large random sample of 4000 men (18–64 yr old) living in central Sweden [11]. A total of 2608 subjects responded to a mailed questionnaire on health, sleep problems in general, and RLS, investigated by means of the four symptom questions determined by the International Restless Legs Syndrome Study Group (IRLSSG). Of the sample, 5.8% suffered from RLS and those with RLS were more likely to report hypertension and heart problems than subjects without (Table 12.1).

Ohayon and Roth used a telephone interview technique with the Sleep-EVAL system across five European countries (UK, Germany, Italy, Portugal, and Spain) to identify factors associated with RLS and periodic limb movement disorder (PLMD) [12]. The sample included 18 980 subjects aged 15–100 years old. The RLS prevalence was 5.5%, significantly increasing with age. Hypertension (treated or not), heart disease, and diabetes were significantly associated with RLS (Table 12.1).

Phillips et al., examining the data from the 2005 National Sleep Foundation Poll in the United States, including 1506 adults as a representative sample of U.S. adults, found that

Table 12.1. Studies on association between restless legs syndrome, hypertension, and cardiovascular diseases

Author	Method	Population	Patients with RLS	Association with CVD
Ulfberg et al., 2001 [11]	Self-reporting questionnaire	4000 men living in Sweden (2608 respondents)	231	RLS sufferers more frequently reported hypertension (OR, 1.5; 95% CI, 0.9–2.4) and heart problems (OR, 2.5; 95% CI, 1.4–4.3)
Ohayon and Roth, 2002 [12]	Telephone interview (Sleep-EVAL system)	18 980 subjects (15–100 yr old) from five European countries	5.5%	Significantly greater percentage of hypertension (OR, 1.36; 95% CI, 1.14–1.61) and heart disease (OR, 1.41; 95% CI, 1.06–1.88) in the RLS population
Berger et al. 2004 [22]	Face-to-face interview (including 4 standardized questions for RLS criteria) and physical examination	Random 4310 participants (20–79 yr old) (Study of Health, Pomerania, northeastern Germany): 4107 subjects included in the analysis	10.6%	Higher prevalence of myocardial infarction among RLS subjects
Foley et al., 2004 [23]	Telephone interview	1506 community-dwelling 55–84 yr-old subjects	10%	Heart disease is associated with unpleasant feelings in legs (OR, 1.68; 95% CI, 1.09–2.57)
Winkelman et al., 2006 [18]	Mailed questionnaire	Random sample of 6569 men and women 30–60 yr old (Wisconsin Sleep Cohort Study): 2821 respondents	300	Daily RLS symptoms are associated with an increased prevalence of CVD (OR, 2.58; 95% CI, 1.38–4.84)
Phillips et al., 2006 [13]	Telephone interview	Random sample of 1506 adults representative of US adults (National Sleep Foundation Poll)	9.7%	The presence of many of the medical conditions including hypertension and heart disease were associated with RLS symptoms (P=0.05 and 0.10, respectively)

Study	Method	Sample	Prevalence	Findings
Winkelman et al., 2008 [19]	Self-administered questionnaire including the 4 International RLS study group diagnostic criteria	3433 adults (Sleep Heart Health Study)	6.8% (women) 3.3% (men)	The associations of RLS with coronary artery disease and CVD were stronger in subjects with RLS symptoms at least 16 times per month and were stronger in those with severe symptoms. OR for coronary artery disease = 2.05, 95% CI,1.38–3.04; OR for CVD = 2.07, 95% CI,1.43–3.00 for subjects with RLS compared to those without RLS
Wesstrom et al., 2008 [20]	Questionnaire	Random sample of 5000 women aged 18–64 yr from Swedish population (response rate: 70.3%)	15.7%	RLS subjects more often suffered from heart disease
Mallon et al., 2008 [14]	Questionnaire	Random sample of 5102 adults from central Sweden (3550 respondents)	885 (25.3%)	Men and women with RLS had more often hypertension and heart disease
Juuti et al., 2010 [24]	Self-administered questionnaires including 4 International RLS study group diagnostic criteria	1332 from unselected 57-year-old urban population in northen Finland (995 participants)	179	Strong and independent positive association between RLS and CVD (OR= 2.92, 95% CI,1.18–7.23).
Benediktsdottir et al., 2010 [21]	Questionnaire including International RLS Rating Scale	Random sample of 1937 adults aged 40+ yr living in Iceland and Sweden (1370 respondents)	18.3% in Iceland; 11.5% in Sweden	RLS was not associated with hypertension or CVD
Möller et al., 2010 [15]	Questionnaire including International RLS Rating Scale	16 531 patients visiting 1 of 312 primary care practices in Germany (mean age: 55 yr)	1758 (10.6%)	Hypertension and heart rate were significantly more prevalent in RLS patients (P<0.0001)

RLS, restless legs syndrome; CVD, cardiovascular diseases.

9.7% of respondents reported symptoms of RLS at least a few nights a week [13]. Other medical conditions, including hypertension and diabetes, were associated with RLS symptoms (P=0.05), and there was a trend (P=0.10) of an association with RLS symptoms in those with heart disease. Several lifestyle factors were also linked with RLS symptoms. In particular, subjects who declared cigarette smoking were more likely to report RLS symptoms (P=0.05) (Table 12.1).

Utilizing the data from 1559 men and 1874 women (mean age of 67.9 years) enrolled in the Sleep Heart Health Study, Winkelman et al. found a higher risk of both coronary artery disease and CVD in the RLS population, after controlling for confounding variables such as age, gender, race, BMI, diabetes, systolic blood pressure, antihypertension medication use, total cholesterol, LDL cholesterol ratio, and smoking history [19]. Patients with moderate to severe RLS had the highest risk for coronary artery disease or cerebrovascular disease (Table 12.1).

Möller et al. studied a large sample of 16 531 patients consulting one of 312 primary care practices in Germany [15]. All patients filled out a self-assessment questionnaire and patients who reported suffering from unpleasant sensations in the legs were then assessed by the physician. A total of 1758 patients (10.6%) were diagnosed with RLS according to the four essential clinical IRLSSG criteria (Table 12.1). Comorbidity rates were significantly higher in RLS patients compared with the control group of patients with other kinds of leg problems. More interestingly, a subanalysis revealed that increased rates of hypertension, diabetes, and heart disease were only evident in RLS patients younger than 60 years of age, indicating that typical illnesses of older age tend to occur earlier in RLS patients [15].

Using the national registries of inhabitants, Benediktsdottir et al. studied a random sample of adults aged 40 years and over, living in Iceland and Sweden, who were invited to participate in a study on the prevalence of chronic obstructive pulmonary disease (COPD) [21]. In addition, the participants were asked to answer the international RLS rating scale questionnaire. Restless legs syndrome was not associated with symptoms of the metabolic syndrome, like hypertension and obesity or CVD, but subjects with RLS were more likely to be ex- and current smokers than subjects without RLS (P<0.001) (Table 12.1).

In summary, the results of the studies suggest a possible relationship between self-reported RLS symptoms, hypertension, and CVD persisting even after adjustment for multiple potential confounders, including age, gender, sleep disorders, BMI, and lifestyle factors. However, a definitive conclusion is elusive because of the difficulties in comparing the results from the studies characterized by high heterogeneity in participants' demographics (age and lifestyle habits), and in the methods used in ascertainments, and definition of hypertension, CVD, and RLS. Not all studies use the established four IRLSSG diagnostic criteria or assessed the frequency of RLS symptoms to differentiate RLS severity and its possible impact on general health. In many studies, the RLS patients were not interviewed or examined to exclude RLS mimics. The definition of hypertension or CVD is sometimes based only on affirmative responses to a single question [3].

Association of restless legs syndrome, hypertension, and cardiovascular diseases: the possible mechanisms

Autonomic activation

Restless legs syndrome may increase the risk of CVD via chronic activation of the sympathetic nervous system with PLMS [25]. A polysomnographic study by Espinar-Sierra et al. on

91 subjects with essential hypertension found that the prevalence of PLM in sleep was directly proportional to the severity of hypertension [26]. Patients with grade III hypertension had a 36.4% prevalence of PLMS, and patients with grade I and II hypertension had a 13% prevalence of PLMS. This relationship was independent of age, gender, obesity, smoking, alcohol consumption, apnea severity, and use of antihypertensive medications [26]. The study conducted by Billars et al. in a much larger population of 861 patients with self-reported RLS symptoms also found that the risk for having hypertension was twice as high for those with a PLMS index of >30 (OR=2.26; 95% CI, 1.28–3.99), independent of other confounding factors [27].

Although the trend for higher daytime blood pressure in children with PLMS was not significant in a recent cross-sectional study involving 314 children, children with PLMS were at significantly higher risk for nocturnal systolic and diastolic hypertension [28].

Increased PLMS rates are frequently observed in patients with congestive heart failure (CHF) and also in heart transplant recipients compared to controls, often independent of concomitant sleep-disordered breathing [29–31].

A number of studies have demonstrated a temporal coincidence between PLMS and pulse rate elevations (Figure 12.3). Pennestri et al. [32], Sforza et al. [33], Ferri et al. [34], and Siddiqui et al. [35] documented significant repetitive systolic and diastolic blood pressure and heart rate (HR) elevations coinciding with PLMS in RLS patients. Heart rate and blood pressure elevations that accompany PLMS occurred whether there was an accompanying EEG arousal, but their magnitude increased in patients in whom EEG microarousals or arousals accompanied the PLMS. Sforza et al. [33] found that there is a hierarchy of arousals accompanying the PLMS, from autonomic activation to bursts of delta activity to alpha

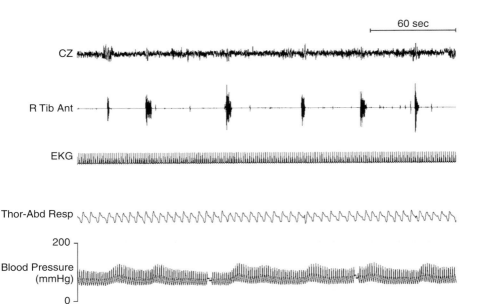

Figure 12.3. Periodic limb movements in a patient with restless legs syndrome. Muscle contractions are associated with evident blood pressure elevations. R Tib Ant, right tibialis anterior muscle; EKG, electrocardiogram; Thor-Abd Resp, thoracoabdominal respirogram.

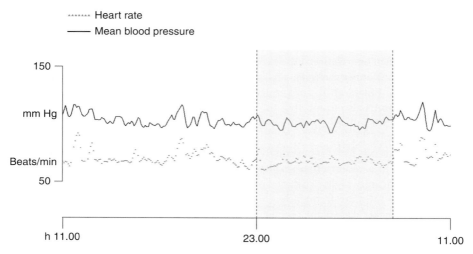

Figure 12.4. Twenty-four-hour mean blood pressure and heart rate recordings in a restless legs syndrome patient. The 24-hour blood pressure profile documented the absence of physiological dipping of blood pressure during the night.

activity to a full awakening. When PLMS were accompanied by theta activity or alpha activity, the HR was even faster [33,36].

Sympathetic activation accompanying PLMS is greater than for all other movement types occurring during sleep, as measured by HR variability spectra [37]. Siddiqui et al. [35] emphasized the importance of the relationship between PLMS and sleep-respiratory events and found a linear correlation between rise in blood pressure and the duration of respiratory-related limb movements.

Recently, Manconi et al. [38] documented that treatment of PLMS with pramipexole reduced the number of PLMSs and the amplitude of the autonomic response to residual PLMS, stressing that normalization of the HR response could be relevant in reducing the risk of developing CVD in patients with RLS.

In summary, the resulting overactivity of the sympathetic nervous system due to PLMS seems to be responsible for the consequent increase in blood pressure variability (Figure 12.4.) The elevations in pulse rates and blood pressure linked to PLMS themselves, or more probably to the arousals associated with PLMS, lead to the development of daytime hypertension and probably increase the risk for subsequent CVD. An alternative explanation is that rises in pulse rate and blood pressure associated with PLMS could cause CVD through an increased risk of atherosclerotic plaque formation and rupture [19]. Considering that one of the leading hypotheses for the pathogenesis of RLS and PLMS is a link to a dopaminergic deficit, Walters and Rye suggest that a spinal dopaminergic hypofunction could manifest as heightened sympathetic efferent drive [25].

Hypothalamic–pituitary–adrenal system overactivity

An overactive HPA system is a possible mechanism contributing to the enhanced load of CVD in RLS patients [39]. Schilling et al. [39] investigated nocturnal urinary cortisol excretion as an indicator of HPA system activity in 73 RLS patients compared with 34 healthy controls matched for age and gender. They found significantly enhanced nocturnal cortisol excretion in RLS, demonstrating nocturnal HPA system overactivity in RLS.

These data were not found in an earlier study, in which Wetter et al. [40] reported no differences in nocturnal cortisol levels. These differences are probably due to the smaller sample size in Wetter's study and the selection of the patients suffering from mild RLS.

Sleep loss

Restless legs syndrome could increase the risk for CVD via its well-documented profound adverse effects on sleep. Sleep loss can also promote glucose intolerance, proinflamatory changes, dyslipidemia, obesity, and hypertension. Although the results of investigations on the effect of sleep deprivation on the daytime blood pressure level of healthy subjects have not always been consistent, different studies seem to indicate that too short sleep duration causes an elevated 24-hour blood pressure and is associated with a higher risk for hypertension and CVD [8,41].

A recent ten-year longitudinal study of 4810 normotensive subjects between the ages of 32 and 59 years documented that those who reported averaging five hours of sleep per night were at an increased risk for developing hypertension over the follow-up period compared to those who routinely had a sleep duration of six to eight hours a night [41]. The authors emphasized that habitually short sleep duration could lead to the development and maintenance of hypertension through prolonged exposure to raised 24-hour blood pressure and heart rate, elevated sympathetic nervous system activity, waking physical and psychosocial stressors, and increased salt retention. The extended exposure to these factors could lead to the entrainment of the cardiovascular system to operate at an elevated pressure equilibrium through structural adaptations, such as arterial and left ventricle hypertrophic remodeling. Chronic short sleep durations could also contribute to hypertension by disrupting circadian rhythmicity and autonomic balance.

Eguchi et al. performed ambulatory blood pressure monitoring in 1255 hypertensive patients (mean age, 70.4 yr) and followed them for a mean period of 50 months [42]. The group with shorter sleep duration (<7.5 hr) had a substantially and significantly higher incidence of CVD (stroke, fatal or nonfatal myocardial infarction, and sudden cardiac death) than the group with normal sleep duration.

Other medical conditions

Most studies, mainly cross-sectional, from different countries have assessed the association of RLS to diabetes or impaired glucose tolerance [3]. Of the 24 studies evaluating this association, four indicated none, seven reported a positive but not significant association, 12 documented significant positive associations, and one reported mixed findings [3]. Although not all studies suggested a positive relationship between RLS and diabetes, the association remains robust even after controlling for age, gender, BMI, smoking, and other potentially confounding factors, including neuropathy in one study [3].

No definitive conclusions emerge from the studies on the relationship between BMI, dyslipidemia, and RLS because differences in the definition of obesity and population characteristics make comparisons across studies difficult [3,43,44].

Affective disorders, including depression and anxiety, are also common in patients with RLS, and can exacerbate sleep impairment and lead to HPA-axis dysregulation and autonomic dysfunction, thus promoting a vicious cycle of adverse physiological and neuroendocrine changes that could determine the development and progression of diabetes, CVD, and related conditions [45].

Adverse lifestyle factors such as smoking could contribute to the association between RLS and CVD. It is interesting to remember that recent studies demonstrated a high prevalence of nocturnal smoking and nocturnal eating in RLS patients as compulsive habit behaviors facilitated by the nocturnal arousals characteristic of RLS [46,47].

Conclusion

Emerging evidence suggests an association between RLS and CVD but definitive conclusions are lacking. The broad differences in ascertainment procedures and diagnostic criteria used for both RLS and CVD among the different studies make a comparison across studies challenging. Moreover, some studies were conducted for other reasons and were not specifically designed to investigate CVD in RLS patients. Most of the data collected were derived from cross-sectional studies, and the lack of prospective studies prevents the determination of any temporal relationship between RLS and CVD, thereby precluding a definitive conclusion.

The increased autonomic activity due to PLMS, the effect of chronic sleep deprivation, and comorbidities associated with RLS/PLMS are all possible factors that predispose RLS patients to heart disease and stroke. However, more research is needed to evaluate the role of RLS and PLMS in increasing cardiovascular risk.

References

1. Allen RP, Picchietti D, Hening WA, et al. Restless legs syndrome: diagnostic criteria, special considerations, and epidemiology. A report from the restless legs syndrome diagnosis and epidemiology workshop at the National Institutes of Health. *Sleep Med* 2003; **4**: 101–19.

2. Allen RP, Walters AS, Montplaisir J, et al. Restless legs syndrome prevalence and impact: REST general population study. *Arch Intern Med* 2005; **165**: 1286–92.

3. Innes KE, Selfe TK, Agarwal P. Prevalence of restless legs syndrome in North American and Western European populations: a systematic review. *Sleep Med* 2011; **12**: 623–34.

4. Lugaresi E, Coccagna G, Gambi D, et al. A propos de quelques manifestations nocturnes myocloniques (nocturnal myoclonus de Symonds). *Rev Neurol* 1966; **115**: 547–55.

5. The International Classification of Sleep Disorders. *Diagnostic and Coding Manual.* 2nd edn. Westchester, IL: American Academy of Sleep Medicine, 2005.

6. Lee SJ, Kim JS, Song IU, et al. Poststroke restless legs syndrome and lesion location: anatomical considerations. *Mov Disord* 2009; **24**: 77–84.

7. Walters AS, Moussouttas M, Siddiqui F, et al. Prevalence of stroke in restless legs syndrome: initial results point to the need for more sophisticated studies. *Open Neurol J* 2010; **4**: 73–7.

8. Portaluppi F, Cortelli P, Calandra Buonaura G, et al. Do restless legs syndrome (RLS) and periodic limb movements of sleep (PLMS) play a role in nocturnal hypertension and increased cardiovascular risk of renally impaired patients? *Chronobiol Int* 2009; **26**: 1206–21.

9. Lindner A, Fornadi K, Lazar AS, et al. Periodic limb movements in sleep are associated with stroke and cardiovascular risk factors in patients with renal failure. *J Sleep Res* 2012; **21**: 297–307.

10. La Manna G, Pizza F, Persici E, et al. Restless legs syndrome enhances cardiovascular risk and mortality in patients with end-stage kidney disease undergoing long-term haemodialysis treatment. *Nephrol Dial Transplant* 2011; **26**: 1976–83.

11. Ulfberg J, Nystrom B, Carter N, et al. Prevalence of restless legs syndrome among men aged 18 to 64 years: an association with somatic disease and neuropsychiatric symptoms. *Mov Disord* 2001; **16**: 1159–63.

12. Ohayon MM, Roth T. Prevalence of restless legs syndrome and periodic limb movement disorder in the general population. *J Psychosom Res* 2002; **53**: 547–54.

13. Phillips B, Hening W, Britz P, et al. Prevalence and correlates of restless legs syndrome: results from the 2005 National Sleep Foundation Poll. *Chest* 2006; **129**: 76–80.

14. Mallon L, Broman JE, Hetta J. Restless legs symptoms with sleepiness in relation to mortality: 20-year follow-up study of a middle-aged Swedish population. *Psychiatry Clin Neurosci* 2008; **62**: 457–63.

15. Möller C, Wetter TC, Köster J, et al. Differential diagnosis of unpleasant sensations in the legs: prevalence of restless legs syndrome in a primary care population. *Sleep Med* 2010; **11**: 161–6.

16. Rothdach AJ, Trenkwalder C, Haberstock J, et al. Prevalence and risk factors of RLS in an elderly population: the MEMO study. Memory and morbidity in Augsburg elderly. *Neurology* 2000; **54**: 1064–8.

17. Hogl B, Kiechl S, Willeit J, et al. Restless legs syndrome: a community-based study of prevalence, severity, and risk factors. *Neurology* 2005; **64**: 1920–4.

18. Winkelman JW, Finn L, Young T. Prevalence and correlates of restless legs syndrome symptoms in the Wisconsin Sleep Cohort. *Sleep Med* 2006; **7**: 545–52.

19. Winkelman JW, Shahar E, Sharief I, et al. Association of restless legs syndrome and cardiovascular disease in the Sleep Heart Health Study. *Neurology* 2008; **70**: 35–42.

20. Wesstrom J, Nilsson S, Sundstrom-Poromaa I, et al. Restless legs syndrome among women: prevalence, co-morbidity and possible relationship to menopause. *Climacteric* 2008; **11**: 422–8.

21. Benediktsdottir B, Janson C, Lindberg E, et al. Prevalence of restless legs syndrome among adults in Iceland and Sweden: lung function, comorbidity, ferritin, biomarkers and quality of life. *Sleep Med* 2010; **11**: 1043–8.

22. Berger K, Luedemann J, Trenkwalder C, et al. Sex and the risk of restless legs syndrome in the general population. *Arch Intern Med* 2004; **164**: 196–202.

23. Foley D, Ancoli-Israel S, Britz P, et al. Sleep disturbances and chronic disease in older adults: results of the 2003 National Sleep Foundation Sleep in America Survey. *J Psychosom Res* 2004; **56**: 497–502.

24. Juuti AK, Läär E, Rajala U, et al. Prevalence and associated factors of restless legs in a 57-year-old urban population in northern Finland. *Acta Neurol Scand* 2010; **122**: 63–9.

25. Walters AS, Rye DB. Review of the relationship of restless legs syndrome and periodic limb movements in sleep to hypertension, heart disease, and stroke. *Sleep* 2009; **32**: 589–97.

26. Espinar-Sierra J, Vela-Bueno A, Luque-Otero M. Periodic leg movements in sleep in essential hypertension. *Psychiatry Clin Neurosci* 1997; **51**: 103–7.

27. Billars L, Hicks A, Bliwise D, et al. Hypertension risk and PLMS in restless legs syndrome. *Sleep* 2007; **30**: A297–8.

28. Wing YK, Zhang J, Ho CK, et al. Periodic limb movement during sleep is associated with nocturnal hypertension in children. *Sleep* 2010; **33**: 759–65.

29. Hanly P, Zuberi-Khokhar N. Periodic limb movements during sleep in patients with congestive heart failure. *Chest* 1996; **109**: 1497–502.

30. Javaheri S. Sleep disorders in systolic heart failure: a prospective study of 100 male patients. The final report. *Int J Cardiol* 2006; **106**: 21–8.

31. Skomro R, Silva R, Alves R, et al. The prevalence and significance of periodic leg movements during sleep in patients with congestive heart failure. *Sleep Breath* 2009; **13**: 43–7.

32. Pennestri MH, Montplaisir J, Colombo R, et al. Nocturnal blood pressure changes in patients with restless legs syndrome. *Neurology* 2007; **68**: 1213–18.

33. Sforza E, Nicolas A, Lavigne G, et al. EEG and cardiac activation during periodic leg movements in sleep: support for a hierarchy of arousal responses. *Neurology* 1999; **52**: 786–91.

34. Ferri R, Zucconi M, Rundo F, et al. Heart rate and spectral EEG changes accompanying periodic and non-periodic leg movements during sleep. *Clin Neurophysiol* 2007; **118**: 438–48.

35. Siddiqui F, Strus J, Ming X, et al. Rise of blood pressure with periodic limb movements in sleep and wakefulness. *Clin Neurophysiol* 2007; **118**: 1923–30.

36. Winkelman JW. The evoked heart rate response to periodic leg movements of sleep. *Sleep* 1999; **22**: 575–80.

37. Guggisberg AG, Hess CW, Mathis J. The significance of the sympathetic nervous system in the pathophysiology of periodic leg movements in sleep. *Sleep* 2007; **30**: 755–66.

38. Manconi M, Ferri R, Zucconi M, et al. Effects of acute dopamine-agonist treatment in restless legs syndrome on heart rate variability during sleep. *Sleep Med* 2011; **12**: 47–55.

39. Schilling C, Schredl M, Strobl P, et al. Restless legs syndrome: evidence for nocturnal hypothalamic-pituitary-adrenal system activation. *Mov Disord* 2010; **25**: 1047–52.

40. Wetter TC, Collado-Seidel V, Oertel H, et al. Endocrine rhythms in patients with restless legs syndrome. *J Neurol* 2002; **249**: 146–51.

41. Gangwisch JE, Heymsfield SB, Boden-Albala B, et al. Short sleep duration as a risk factor for hypertension: analyses of the first National Health and Nutrition Examination Survey. *Hypertension* 2006; **47**: 833–9.

42. Eguchi K, Pickering TG, Schwartz JE, et al. Short sleep duration as an independent predictor of cardiovascular events in Japanese patients with hypertension. *Arch Intern Med* 2008; **168**: 2225–31.

43. Schlesinger I, Erikh I, Avizohar O, et al. Cardiovascular risk factors in restless legs syndrome. *Mov Disord* 2009; **24**: 1587–92.

44. Cosentino FII, Aricò D, Lanuzza B, et al. Absence of cardiovascular disease risk factors in restless legs syndrome. *Acta Neurol Scand* 2012; **125**: 319–25.

45. Hornyak M. Depressive disorders in restless legs syndrome: epidemiology, pathophysiology and management. *CNS Drugs* 2010; **24**: 89–98.

46. Provini F, Antelmi E, Vignatelli L, et al. Increased prevalence of nocturnal smoking in restless legs syndrome (RLS). *Sleep Med* 2010; **11**: 218–20.

47. Provini F, Antelmi E, Vignatelli L, et al. Association of restless legs syndrome with nocturnal eating: a case-control study. *Mov Disord* 2009; **24**: 871–7.

Chapter 13

Physician as patient
A personal story of stroke

Harold R. Smith

Prelude

Approximately five years before my stroke, my best friend asked me to start running with him so that he could have a running training partner and we could both train for long-distance running competitions. Prior to joining my friend's running exercise, all of my running experience had been limited to short-distance speed running such as track and field sprint running or sprinting within sports such as football, baseball, or basketball. It quickly became apparent to both of us that I was still running in speed and sprint pacing and that I needed to reset my pacing to long-distance running, which is more to do with stamina than sprint pacing. I began to look for a running road race that was near my home and was being run for good charitable reasons and I found a 10-kilometer charity run that was nearby and was being used as a fund raiser race for an excellent medical support system.

First movement

The 10-km race turned out to be, in my opinion, much more of a speed race than a long-distance stamina race.

I was placed first in the 10-km race for my age group. The race finished in front of a race sponsoring an athletic supplies store. Employees of the store approached me after my first-place finish and informed me that my running time for the 10-km victory was of a speed that would be representative of an established competitive runner and they asked me if I would join the athletic supplies store running team. I trained with this team for several months.

Second movement

The entire running team with whom I was now training enrolled in another 10-km charity race in a different locale. In this second race I was again placed first for my age group, and as I was completing my first-place finish, I passed and left behind a member of my running team who had been an Olympic medalist for this length of running race in the past. This team member suggested to me that I consider becoming a full-time runner for both speed runs and long-distance running.

Sleep, Stroke, and Cardiovascular Disease, ed. Antonio Culebras. Published by Cambridge University Press. © Cambridge University Press 2013.

Third movement

I returned to long-distance running training with my best friend and learned to change my pacing, running form, and running strategy to be more appropriate for long-distance stamina runs, and this retraining turned out to be very successful in that I was placed first for my age group in the first charity half-marathon in which I competed. All of my running training and competition had resulted in me being extraordinarily healthy, fit, and active compared to all other men in my age group. My internal medicine physicians encouraged me to continue with my running in that they felt that my health profile revealed no risk factors for stroke or heart disease because of my running and training. I continued my training runs wherever I traveled. Ironically, even though my friend started my running and training exercise program, he and I never simultaneously participated in a race; we both translated the fitness we gained into mountaineering and deep wilderness hiking and camping exercise.

Fourth movement

I continued my training runs in cities wherever one of my professional medical associations was holding an annual meeting. However, the location of one of these cities did not have the hilly terrain that is required for one of my usual training runs. I had learned previously how consolidated my sleep had been when I was able to continue the run and training regimen. Thus, in contrast to when I was not able to complete that training run because of the inappropriate terrain, I quickly developed nonconsolidated sleep. My writing of these recollections helped me to understand the occurrence of a seemingly contradictory health catastrophe such as my stroke occurring in a man more fit and active than virtually any other man the same age. If the reader will allow me to, I would like to continue what may seem to be a repetitious recounting of past athletic victorious competitions and the training leading thereto. This is to explore further and to understand how my stroke survival and recovery resulted in such rapid and remarkable advances in physical activities, like recovery of ambulation, bed and chair transfers, and balance, that were ahead of my fellow stroke survivors' recoveries because my prestoke strength and discipline were so well developed relative to theirs. While in the regimen of training, when I missed one training run in the annual meeting city I had, for the first time in many years, a night with poorly consolidated sleep.

Coda

When I returned home from the annual meeting city and I resumed my normal training regimen, my sleep returned to the consolidated pattern that I had in the past when I was able to continue an uninterrupted pattern of training runs.

I volunteered to be a control subject in a sleep study project at my center for sleep medicine. During that sleep study my sleep was interrupted frequently by monitoring equipment alarms sounding because of very low resting heart rates (my heart rate at rest was normally in the 30–40 beats/min range due to my running regimens). These frequent extrinsic arousals from sleep resulted in nonconsolidated sleep very uncharacteristic for me when I was able to maintain my normal exercise patterns. When the sleep study recorded arousals were carefully reviewed later, it was found that the arousals were related exclusively to extrinsic alarm sounds and clearly revealed no intrinsic sleep disorder at all.

The following morning after the sleep study was completed I returned home where I consumed a normal prerun breakfast followed by my normal warm-up and stretching regimen before leaving for a run. I had missed my normal hilly terrain run the preceding week while I was at the annual meeting city. Now that I was home and had easy access to a 19-mile hill and canyon terrain, I embarked on my usual once-monthly hill and canyon run. In all of the years that I was training or competing in runs of any category, I had always used an athletic heart rate monitor to maximize running efficiency and to have data on heart rates so as to be able to replicate heart rates in competitive racing to match the heart rates in maximal efficiency training runs. During my usual once-monthly 19-mile hill and canyon training run, I glanced at my heart rate monitor and read a displayed figure of 108. I became transiently befuddled in that I knew that my heart rate for a 19-mile hill and canyon run could not possibly be that high . As the heart rate monitor continued on to display a read-out of 112, I finally realized that the numbers displayed were not heart rates at that time but rather the display was showing a 1 min 8 s or 1 min 12 s interval time from the start of the run to the location in the run where I was looking at the monitor display. Because I had been transiently befuddled about the monitor displays, which I had never previously experienced at any time, I realized that something was seriously wrong and I chose to return home walking. I am still uncertain how I managed to walk home through 19 miles of hills and canyons and how I managed to cross two very busy streets that, even without the stroke, are difficult to cross safely. When I returned to my home I explained to my wife what had happened and that I felt that something was seriously wrong. My wife, who holds R. N. and BSN degrees, measured my blood pressure at 130/70 – which is a blood pressure that I had remained at steadily for several decades. She immediately stated that she felt that I was showing signs of having had a stroke and she called for paramedics. When the paramedics arrived they indicated that their plan was to transport me to a trauma center hospital. I argued with the paramedics and demanded to be taken to the hospital with a stroke center unit (I had helped to form the stroke unit at the hospital one year earlier). At the stroke center I was rapidly diagnosed and successfully treated for a right internal carotid artery dissection. One of the treatment team physicians commented to me that the dissection such as I had may occur in athletic people performing their normal athletic activities and the dissection did not require any independent or additional trauma to occur. One of my former students working at the stroke unit asked me about any known sleep disorders that I may have.

The beginning of the end

I explained to my former student that I had no known sleep disorders at all, in fact I had been part of a sleep study the night preceding the stroke, which showed numerous extrinsic arousals due to medical equipment alarms. These extrinsic arousals disrupted my sleep architecture and disturbed my sleep consolidation. In retrospect, I believe that the numerous intrinsic sleep disorders per se that patients may have may not be the primary risk factor for stroke or heart disease but rather the arousals and associated disrupted sleep architecture that is caused by these disorders, or any other cause of frequent arousal or disruption of normal sleep consolidation, may be the more proximate risk factor for stroke and heart disease, and should be taken into account in all investigations. I suggest that the arousal index and disrupted sleep architecture should be considered when methodologically evaluating risk-factor relationships of sleep and sleep disorder with stroke and cardiovascular disease. Additionally, for persons who have arousals that occur due to extrinsic disruptions such as I had with medical equipment alarms, or patients whose bed partners interrupt their sleep due to activities such as loud snoring, restlessness, or similar such disturbances, these extrinsic factors may eventually result in "secondary or second-hand stroke," to coin a term.

If I may change my recollection focus briefly, I would like to remind our readers of the years, not so long ago, in which stroke survivors were treated in "rehab." modalities such as physical therapy, occupational therapy, speech therapy, etc., in the same facility and unit in which their acute stroke diagnosis and initial treatment occurred. This continuity of location and care very importantly also results in continuity of their stroke treatment team as well, which assures that important points of history, examination, testing, and treatment remain clear for uninterrupted continuity of care. In my personal experience, following my transfer to a "stroke rehab. hospital" from my acute care stroke hospital, I was informed by the "rehab. hospital"'s doctor that I was going to be treated with a stimulant medication for the purpose of "doing what we tell you to do." I reminded the doctor that I had recently survived a catastrophic right internal carotid artery dissection and stroke and that we should reconsider adding stimulant medication into that cumulative neurological *gestalt* at the time of his recommendation.

My progress (without stimulant medication) in physical therapy compared to that of my fellow stroke survivors was so rapid while in the "rehab. hospital" that I was often used as an example to these fellow patients: "Do it like Dr. Smith does." This resulted in much grumbling and disparagement aimed in my direction by the other patients (e.g., "If I was a runner like Dr. Smith was then maybe I could walk, transfer, and balance like him").

Further personal experiences at the "rehab. hospital" included being astonished at the hostility aimed at any "rehab. patient" seeking to sleep. In fact, any of the "rehab. patients" who had the temerity to take a daytime nap had their feet taken by the unit staff and placed on the cold floor followed by a forceful transfer to a wheelchair that was moved to the intersection of two walls in the corner of the patient's room. In addition, a stern admonishment followed in the gist of "If you think you should sleep, you might want to reconsider during this time-out in the corner of the room." It is obvious that stroke and cardiovascular, and rehabilitation specialists need thorough and careful continuing medical education efforts about the importance of sleep and sleep disorders in the health and the recovery of all patients.

One further personal experience that prompts my emphasis on continuity of care for acute and "rehab." stroke and cardiovascular patients occurred when my complaints to "rehab." staff of lower extremity discomfort and difficulties with efforts of breathing were ignored. Perhaps those acute care physicians who had recent knowledge by medical history that the patient was a long-distance runner who routinely trained 50 plus miles per week and who was now confined to strict bed rest would have considered initiating evaluation and treatment for stasis/deep vein thrombosis before two massive pulmonary emboli occurred. The pulmonary emboli effectively ended any hope of subsequent return to any sort of stamina-related exercise and/or athletics and very nearly ended my return to any life activities of any sort, as was pointed out by my intensive care unit physicians when the "rehab. hospital" physicians decided that a transfer back to the acute care hospital was in order. We all must now await future chapters, if any.

Index